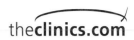

CRITICAL CARE NURSING CLINICS OF NORTH AMERICA

Sedation and Sleep in Critical Care

GUEST EDITOR
Jan Foster, PhD, RN, CNS, CCRN, CCN

CONSULTING EDITOR
Suzanne S. Prevost, PhD, RN, CNAA

September 2005 • Volume 17 • Number 3

SAUNDERS

An Imprint of Elsevier, Inc.
PHILADELPHIA   LONDON   TORONTO   MONTREAL   SYDNEY   TOKYO

W.B. SAUNDERS COMPANY
A Division of Elsevier Inc.

Elsevier Inc., 1600 John F. Kennedy Blvd., Suite 1800, Philadelphia, PA 19103-2899.

http://www.theclinics.com

CRITICAL CARE NURSING CLINICS OF NORTH AMERICA   Volume 17, Number 3
September 2005   ISSN 0899-5885
Editor: Maria Lorusso   ISBN 1-4160-2652-5

Reprints. For copies of 100 or more, of articles in this publication, please contact the Commercial Reprints Department, Elsevier Inc., 360 Park Avenue South, New York, New York 10010-1710. Tel. (212) 633-3813 Fax: (212) 462-1935 e-mail: reprints@elsevier.com

The ideas and opinions expressed in *Critical Care Nursing Clinics of North America* do not necessarily reflect those of the Publisher. The Publisher does not assume any responsibility for any injury and/or damage to persons or property arising out of or related to any use of the material contained in this periodical. The reader is advised to check the appropriate medical literature and the product information currently provided by the manufacturer of each drug to be administered to verify the dosage, the method and duration of administration, or contraindications. It is the responsibility of the treating physician or other health care professional, relying on independent experience and knowledge of the patient, to determine drug dosages and the best treatment for the patient. Mention of any product in this issue should not be construed as endorsement by the contributors, editors, or the Publisher of the product or manufacturers' claims.

Critical Care Nursing Clinics of North America (ISSN 0899-5885) is published quarterly by W.B. Saunders Company. Corporate and editorial offices: Elsevier Inc., 1600 John F. Kennedy Blvd., Suite 1800, Philadelphia, PA 19103-2899. Accounting and circulation offices: 6277 Sea Harbor Drive, Orlando, FL 32887-4800. Periodicals postage paid at Orlando, FL 32862, and additional mailing offices. Subscription prices are $100.00 per year for US individuals, $164.00 per year for US institutions, $70.00 per year for US students and residents, $132.00 per year for Canadian individuals, $203.00 per year for Canadian institutions, $140.00 per year for international individuals, $203.00 per year for international institutions and $70.00 per year for Canadian and foreign students/residents. To receive student/resident rate, orders must be accompanied by name of affiliated institution, date of term, and the *signature* of program/residency coordinator on institution letterhead. Orders will be billed at individual rate until proof of status is received. Foreign air speed delivery is included in all *Clinics* subscription prices. All prices are subject to change without notice. POSTMASTER: Send address changes to *Critical Care Nursing Clinics of North America,* W.B. Saunders Company, Periodicals Fulfillment, Orlando, FL 32887-4800. **Customer Service: 1-800-654-2452 (US). From outside of the US, call 1-407-345-4000.**

Critical Care Nursing Clinics of North America is covered in *International Nursing Index, Nursing Citation Index, Cumulative Index to Nursing and Allied Health Literature, and RNdex Top 100.*

Printed in the United States of America.

GOAL STATEMENT

The goal of *Critical Care Nursing Clinics of North America* is to keep practicing critical care nurses up to date with current critical care clinical practice by providing timely articles reviewing the state of the art in critical care.

ACCREDITATION

The *Critical Care Nursing Clinics of North America* is planned and implemented in accordance with the Essential Areas and Policies of the Accreditation Council for Continuing Medical Education (ACCME) through the joint sponsorship of the University of Virginia School of Medicine and Elsevier. The University of Virginia School of Medicine is accredited by the ACCME to provide continuing medical education for physicians.

The University of Virginia School of Medicine designates this educational activity for a maximum of 60 category 1 credits per year, 15 category 1 credits per issue, toward the AMA Physician's Recognition Award. Each practitioner should claim only those credits that he/she actually spent in the activity. *NOTE: The American Nurses Credentialing Center (ANCC), and many State Boards accept AMA category 1 credit issued by an ACCME provider to maintain ANA certifications or licensure. 15 AMA category 1 credits are equivalent to 18 ANA contact hours.*

Category 1 credit can be earned by reading the text material, taking the CME examination online at http://www.theclinics.com/home/cme, and completing the evaluation. After taking the test, you will be required to review any and all incorrect answers. Following completion of the test and evaluation, your credit will be awarded and you may print your certificate.

FACULTY DISCLOSURE

As a provider accredited by the Accreditation Council for Continuing Medical Education (ACCME), the Office of Continuing Medical Education of the University of Virginia School of Medicine must ensure balance, independence, objectivity, and scientific rigor in all its individually sponsored or jointly sponsored educational activities. All authors/editors participating in a sponsored activity are expected to disclose to the readers any significant financial interest or other relationship (1) with the manufacturer(s) of any commercial product(s) and/or provider(s) of commercial services discussed in an educational presentation and (2) with any commercial supporters of the activity (significant financial interest or other relationship can include such things as grants or research support, employee, consultant, stock holder, member of speakers bureau, etc.) The intent of this disclosure is not to prevent authors/editors with a significant financial or other relationship from writing an article, but rather to provide readers with information on which they can make their own judgments. It remains for the readers to determine whether the author's/editor's interest or relationships may influence the article with regard to exposition or conclusion.

The authors/editors listed below have identified no professional or financial affiliations related to their presentation:
Margaret-Ann Carno, PhD, MBA, RNC, CCRN; Heidi V. Connolly, MD; Michael W. Day, MSN, RN, CCRN; Janet G. Whetstone, Foster, PhD, RN, CNS, CCRN; Carmelo Graffagnino, MD, MS; Roberta Kaplow, PhD, RN, CCNS, CCRN; Kenneth J. King, BSN, RN; Melissa A. Miller, PharmD; DaiWai M. Olson, BSN, RN, CCRN; Carol A. Puz, RN, MS, CCRN; Judith L. Reishtein, PhD, RN, CCRN; Pam Sheldon, RN, NREMT; Debora Simmons, MSN, RN,CCRN, CCNS; Brian S. Smith, PharmD; Sandra J. Stokes, MSN, RN; Dinesh Yogaratnam, PharmD; and, Antonia Zapantis, PharmD, MS.

Disclosure of discussion of non-FDA approved uses for pharmaceutical products and/or medical devices: The University of Virginia School of Medicine, as an ACCME provider, requires that all authors/editors identify and disclose any "off label" uses for pharmaceutical products and/or for medical devices. The University of Virginia School of Medicine recommends that each reader fully review all the available data on new products or procedures prior to instituting them with patients.

The authors/editors listed below have not provided disclosure or off-label information:
Simon Leung, PharmD and John Lynch, MD.

TO ENROLL

To enroll in the Critical Care Nursing Clinics of North America Continuing Medical Education program, call customer service at 1-800-654-2452 or sign up online at **http://www.theclinics.com/home/cme**. The CME program is available to subscribers for an additional annual fee of $XXX.00.

GUEST EDITOR

JAN FOSTER, PhD, RN, CNS, CCRN, CCN, Assistant Professor, College of Nursing, Texas Woman's University, Houston; and Nursing Inquiry and Intervention, The Woodlands, Texas

CONTRIBUTORS

MARGARET-ANN CARNO, PhD, MBA, RNC, CCRN, Assistant Professor of Nursing and Pediatrics, University of Rochester School of Nursing, Rochester, New York

HEIDI V. CONNOLLY, MD, Assistant Professor of Pediatrics, Pediatric Critical Care and Sleep Medicine, University of Rochester, Rochester, New York

MICHAEL W. DAY, RN, MSN, CCRN, Outreach Educator/Clinical Nurse Specialist, Northwest MedStar, Spokane, Washington

JAN FOSTER, PhD, RN, CNS, CCRN, CCN, Assistant Professor, College of Nursing, Texas Woman's University, Houston; and Nursing Inquiry and Intervention, The Woodlands, Texas

CARMELO GRAFFAGNINO, MD, FRCPC, Associate Clinical Professor of Medicine–Neurology; and Director, Neuroscience Intensive Care Unit, Department of Internal Medicine, Duke University Medical Center, Durham, North Carolina

CHERYL KABELI, FNP, Cardiothoracic Nurse Practitioner and Clinical Nurse Specialist, Department of Cardiology, Champlain Valley Physicians Hospital, Plattsburgh, New York

ROBERTA KAPLOW, RN, PhD, AOCNS, CCNS, CCRN, Clinical Professor, Nell Hodgson Woodruff School of Nursing, Emory University, Atlanta, Georgia

KENNETH KING, RN, BSN, Staff Nurse, Duke University Medical Center, Durham, North Carolina

SIMON LEUNG, MS, PharmD, Assistant Professor of Pharmacy Practice, College of Pharmacy, Nova Southeastern University, Ft. Lauderdale; and Clinical Pharmacist, Department of Pharmacy, Cleveland Clinic Hospital, Weston, Florida

JOHN R. LYNCH, MD, Assistant Professor of Medicine–Neurology, Department of Internal Medicine, Duke University Medical Center, Durham, North Carolina

MELISSA A. MILLER, PharmD, Pharmacy Practice Resident, Department of Pharmacy, University of Massachusetts Memorial Medical Center, Worcester, Massachusetts

DAIWAI M. OLSON, RN, BSN, CCRN, Doctoral Student, The University of North Carolina at Chapel Hill, School of Nursing, Chapel Hill; and Staff Nurse, Duke University Medical Center, Durham, North Carolina

CAROL A. PUZ, RN, MS, CCRN, Education and Development Specialist, Critical Care, The Western Pennsylvania Hospital, Pittsburgh, Pennsylvania

JUDITH L. REISHTEIN, PhD, RN, Post Doctoral Fellow, School of Nursing and Center for Sleep and Respiratory Neurobiology, University of Pennsylvania, Philadelphia, Pennsylvania

PAM SHELDON, RN, NREMT, Director of Operations, Northwest MedStar, Spokane, Washington

DEBORA SIMMONS, RN, MSN, CCRN, CCNS, The Institute for Healthcare Excellence, The University of Texas MD Anderson Cancer Center, Houston, Texas

BRIAN S. SMITH, PharmD, BCPS, Clinical Pharmacy Specialist–Critical Care Surgery and Trauma, Department of Pharmacy, University of Massachusetts Memorial Medical Center, Worcester, Massachusetts

SANDRA J. STOKES, RN, MSN, Education and Development Specialist, The Western Pennsylvania Hospital, Pittsburgh, Pennsylvania

DINESH YOGARATNAM, PharmD, Clinical Pharmacy Specialist–Critical Care, Department of Pharmacy, University of Massachusetts Memorial Medical Center, Worcester, Massachusetts

ANTONIA ZAPANTIS, MS, PharmD, Assistant Professor of Pharmacy, Department of Pharmacy Practice, College of Pharmacy, Nova Southeastern University, Ft. Lauderdale; and Clinical Education Coordinator, Department of Pharmacy, North Broward Medical Center, Weston, Florida

CONTENTS

increase in morbidity and mortality in patients with obstructive sleep apnea when they are administered anesthesia in conjunction with sedation. There are few reports of sedation alone and obstructive sleep apnea; most studies have been in relation to anesthesia, surgery, patient-controlled analgesia, and sleep-disordered breathing.

FORTHCOMING ISSUES

RECENT ISSUES

THE CLINICS ARE NOW AVAILABLE ONLINE!

Access your subscription at:
www.theclinics.com

CRITICAL CARE
NURSING CLINICS
OF NORTH AMERICA

Crit Care Nurs Clin N Am 17 (2005) xiii – xiv

Preface

Sedation and Sleep in Critical Care

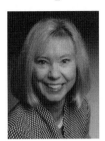

Jan Foster, PhD, RN, CNS, CCRN, CCN
Guest Editor

Sedation is a necessary component of care for critically ill and injured individuals. Sedatives assist in coping with mechanical ventilation and other invasive devices, and help patients tolerate procedures and noxious stimuli in the intensive care unit. Sedatives are also useful in the control of agitation and delirium. In addition to fundamental humane reasons, calming patients with sedatives provides physiologic benefits, such as reducing oxygen consumption expended during restlessness, and prevents dislodgement of life-preserving tubes and catheters. When administering sedatives to manage critically ill patients, clinicians must be cognizant of the many complex issues surrounding their use.

In this issue, Zapantis describes the problems of tolerance and withdrawal of sedatives in critical care. Nurses are frequently challenged with weaning patients from sedation, which necessitates a balance between providing adequate sedation to control agitation, often confounded by withdrawal symptoms. Titrating doses to achieve a state of calm while discontinuing sedatives requires vigilance and knowledge of drug properties. Hepatic and renal function can influence patient responses, dosing requirements, and further challenge the weaning process. Yogaratnam provides an in-depth look at the effects of liver and renal dysfunction on the pharmacokinetics of sedatives and analgesics and the impact on critically ill patients.

Assessment of patients' level of sedation assists in determining progress toward the achievement of the goals of sedation, particularly when sedatives are given primarily for agitation and restlessness. Numerous subjective instruments have been developed for this purpose with varying degrees of proved validity and reliability. None have been perfected for all patient needs, however, and are especially problematic when evaluating neurologic response in brain-injured individuals. Olson describes the use of bispectral analysis, an objective instrument, in evaluating neurologic status in patients receiving sedation. Although particularly problematic in neurologically impaired patients, difficulty gauging appropriate sedation level in all patients may contribute to oversedation. Patients are at risk for prolonged immobility and numerous related complications as a result of the illness or injury, which are compounded by oversedation. Foster discusses the synergistic effect of critical illness and sedation-related problems faced in the acute period and interference with long-term recovery following critical illness.

Sheldon and Day provide a look at sedation issues unique to transportation of critically ill and injured patients, both from crash site to hospital and interhospital transport. They address the various sedation needs of this patient population and challenges for caregivers. Another population with sedation needs is patients experiencing alcohol withdrawal, which can be life-threatening. Puz describes an instrument for use in assessment of alcohol withdrawal to treat patients timely and adequately to prevent serious complications.

Safety is a topic of great concern in hospitals all across the nation. In Simmons' article, she describes a model used for a system-wide approach to problem identification and solutions. Using this model, health care organizations are able to change from a punitive to a safety enhanced culture.

Sleep disruption in critically ill patients is highly underreported, arises from numerous sources, and can interfere with the therapeutic regimen. Critically ill cancer patients report sleep disorders caused by the effects of chemotherapy, bioimmune responses, disturbance in circadian rhythms, and pain, for example. In this issue, Kaplow synthesizes a comprehensive review of the literature on sleep deprivation unique to acutely and critically ill cancer patients and psychosocial impacts. Critically ill children have special growth and development needs affected by illness and potentially further neglected by disorganized sleep patterns. Carno reports numerous sleep and sedation issues experienced by children in the pediatric intensive care unit. Finally, in Reishtein's article, she describes patients' reports of sleep disturbances while receiving mechanical ventilation support.

Jan Foster, PhD, RN, CNS, CCRN, CCN
Texas Woman's University
College of Nursing
1130 John Freeman Boulevard
Houston, TX 77030, USA
E-mail address: jfoster@twu.edu

ELSEVIER
SAUNDERS

Crit Care Nurs Clin N Am 17 (2005) 205 – 210

CRITICAL CARE
NURSING CLINICS
OF NORTH AMERICA

Sedation Issues in Transportation of Acutely and Critically Ill Patients

Pam Sheldon, RN, NREMT, Michael W. Day, RN, MSN, CCRN*

Northwest MedStar, PO Box 11005, Spokane, WA 99211–1005, USA

Although much has been written in recent years regarding sedation for critically ill and injured patients in general, there is a paucity of evidence regarding sedation in the prehospital or interfacility transportation setting. The use of sedation in ground and air medical transportation requires an understanding of the issues specific to transportation situations. There are commonalities in patient care in ground and air medical transportation and the traditional critical care setting. There are instances, however, in which the use of sedation may be required for both patient management and medical crew and vehicle operational safety [1].

Impact on patient care

Patients requiring prehospital transportation to a tertiary care facility are often severely ill or injured and are usually transported directly from the scene. They may be suffering from a variety of traumatic or medical conditions that may require sedation including but not limited to decreased level of consciousness requiring advanced airway management; pain from trauma or medical conditions; anxiety related to the injury or illness; chemical intoxification with substances, such as alcohol, cocaine, methamphetamine, or phencyclidine; or behavior-related issues. Often several conditions coexist and may require detailed evaluation or stabilization at a tertiary care facility. In the prehospital situation, medical trans-

portation crew members may have limited information on the underlying conditions requiring sedation; however, they must appreciate and address the impact of the conditions on the patient's immediate response. Additionally, the patient may require painful or stressful procedures, necessitating sedation. Transportation and the surrounding circumstances are inherently stressful [2,3].

Like prehospital, interfacility transportation is often necessary for acutely and critically ill or traumatized patients to a tertiary care facility for definitive care. In addition to the needs for sedation previously noted, the patient may also have undergone procedures at the referring care facility (surgery, intubation, mechanical ventilation, thoracostomy, and so forth) that require administration of sedatives and analgesics.

In both prehospital and interfacility transportation situations, one of the most important considerations is the patient's mental status and the capacity for airway protection. Establishment and maintenance of a patent airway is always the first priority in care [3]. If a patient is unable to maintain a patent airway from whatever cause, the medical transportation crew members must establish and secure an artificial airway. This is especially important in patients with traumatic brain injuries [4] or compromised ventilation or oxygenation secondary to airway obstruction, hypoventilation, apnea, or flail chest, for example, resulting in hypercapnia or, hypoxemia [5]. Endotracheal intubation provides an avenue for positive pressure ventilation that may not be effective using a bag-valve-mask. Positive pressure ventilation provides for the effective management of both hypercapnia and hypoxemia. In the patient with a flail

* Corresponding author.
E-mail address: daym@nwmedstar.org (M.W. Day).

chest, intubation is considered the definitive therapy because it removes the patient's need to generate negative and positive pressures within the chest wall [5].

In a patient who is not fully conscious, definitive airway management typically entails the use of rapid sequence intubation (RSI). Although there are a number of RSI schemata available, sedation followed by chemical paralysis with a short-acting neuromuscular blocking agent is common before endotracheal intubation. In rare situations in which medical transport crew members are unable successfully to insert an endotracheal tube and the patient cannot be adequately ventilated using a bag-valve-mask device, a cricothyroidotomy becomes necessary, requiring further sedation and analgesia.

In patients with traumatic brain injury, the endotracheal tube is sometimes used to facilitate careful hyperventilation. When signs and symptoms of increased intracranial pressure appear (decreasing level of consciousness, changes in pupillary response, posturing) [4], careful hyperventilation with a resuscitator bag is initiated. A PCO_2 ranging from 32 to 35 torr causes a slight constriction of the cerebral blood vessels, inducing a brief decrease in the increased intracranial pressure. Intravenous mannitol may be administered to maintain decreased intracranial pressure [6].

In addition to sedation, pain management is important in the transportation setting. Patients transported from a prehospital setting or referring facility may experience pain from a variety of sources, including trauma; surgery; procedures; or medical conditions, such as myocardial infarction. The most common pain medications used in transport (morphine, fentanyl, meperidine) also provide some level of sedation. In most instances, added sedation from the analgesia is beneficial. In some situations, however, such as a head trauma, additional sedation may confound the neurologic assessment.

Patients in need of emergent transportation commonly experience anxiety. Anxiety can trigger and result from catecholamine release, which may exacerbate the condition and its associated pain. Sedatives, such as midazolam and lorazepam, act synergistically with opiates and may be useful adjuncts for treatment of anxiety associated with the patient's underlying medical conditions or conditions necessitating transport. An anxiolytic, such as lorazepam, may relax the patient sufficiently and contribute to pain control.

Chemical intoxification by both "street" and prescription drugs is associated with a number of medical conditions and may be a contributing factor of traumatic injury. Chemical intoxification may cause either somnolence or agitation. Decreased level of consciousness, as associated with somnolence from various drugs, may require sedation and intubation to maintain a patent airway and effective ventilation. Some drugs, such as cocaine, methamphetamine, and phencyclidine, cause significant changes in mental status, such as hyperawareness, paranoia, agitation, and violent behavior. Sedation may be required simply to counteract these effects. In many situations, however, the drugs the patient ingested require that they be intubated to protect the airway [7]. In extreme violent behavior, the patient must be sedated to the point where they require intubation, simply for the protection of patient and transportation medical crew members [1,8].

Behavioral issues associated with psychiatric disease can be seen as a comorbidity of the patient' medical condition or traumatic injuries. Assessment of such behavioral issues usually involves determining the cause of the behavior. Examples of such behaviors include affective liability, loud speech, intimidating behaviors, or hostile or aggressive statements. Treatment of such behavioral issues usually involves escalating approaches, from the least to more aggressive [8]. Medical transport crew members may lack the appropriate information to be able to distinguish between psychiatric disease and the other causes of abnormal behavior described previously, such as drug ingestion. In any event, they are almost never in a situation in which they are able to establish a therapeutic client-therapist relationship with the patient. Unfortunately, they are often in the uncomfortable situation of attempting to control the observed behavior. If the observed behavior is of such severity as to threaten either the patient's or crew members' safety, they are usually required by their protocols to sedate the patient to the level where the behavior is no longer a threat [1,9] or refuse to transport the patient. Benzodiazepines are usually recommended for behavioral control issues. Physical restraints, in addition to sedation, are also used for both patient and medical transportation crew members' safety [1,9,10].

In the transportation setting, sedation and pain management may be necessary for the patient's condition [5] and procedures needed to treat the patient. An example is the use of intraosseous devices to deliver fluid or medications emergently. In the adult patient, one type of intraosseous device is placed directly into the manubrium of the sternum. In the pediatric patient, the device is usually placed into the proximal tibia. Because these are often used as a last resort and are usually essential to resuscitate or stabilize the patient, sedation may be required to prevent the patient from dislodging the device.

Transportation mode considerations

Advanced life support transportation generally refers to providing care to patients who are transported from the prehospital setting to a tertiary care facility. Critical care transportation generally refers to an equivalent level of care found in a critical care unit. Many critical care transport services also provide prehospital scene response and may see patients in both arenas of care.

In the United States, the emergency medical services office in the state in which they operate licenses both advanced life support and critical care transportation services. There are some differences between states, but generally paramedics (emergency medical technicians and paramedics) staff the advanced life support transportation services and registered nurses staff the critical care transportation services. There are additional variations of the crew configuration, which may include emergency medical technicians, respiratory care providers, and physicians. The scope of practice for emergency medical technicians and paramedics limits the number and type of medications they are able to administer, unless they have completed additional training to be considered a critical care transportation provider. Registered nurses have a wider knowledge base and experience in dealing with the various drugs seen in the intrafacility transportation setting. Any discussion of a transportation services' ability to use various medications for sedation is entirely dependent on that program's protocols, as established by its medical director, under the specific laws of the states in which it operates. Most advanced life support and critical care transport services operate under protocols that are established and reviewed on a frequent basis by the agency's medical directors. State emergency medical services agencies generally provide direction, but as a rule, allow the medical directors to have a great deal of flexibility and latitude with regard to the use of sedation by their program's medical transportation crew members.

In the prehospital setting, the transportation mode is influenced by a number of factors, including initial agency response capability (basic, intermediate, and advanced life support); distance from the appropriate tertiary medical facility; availability of air medical services; and weather. All of these factors are taken into consideration when a decision is made to transport a patient from a scene. For example, a local basic life support ground unit may transport a patient who is injured in a motor vehicle crash. On a different day, an air medical helicopter may transport a patient with the same injuries from the same location, depending on some of the factors listed previously.

From the interfacility perspective, the referring physician always has the legal responsibility of determining both the most appropriate mode and crew configuration of the transporting agency in relation to the patient's needs. This legal responsibility was established by the Emergency Medical Treatment and Active Labor Act legislation passed by Congress in 1996 [6]. In both the prehospital and interfacility patient transportation, the patient is subject to the additional stress of the transportation, whether by ground or air.

The limitations of transporting a patient in a ground unit typically include space and safe patient access issues while the vehicle is moving. The vibration and swaying (both side-to-side and front-to-back) of a moving vehicle makes it difficult effectively to assess the patient and safely do more than simple interventions. In addition, in the prehospital transportation, it is often difficult to obtain a detailed understanding of the patient's injuries or medical condition. In an aircraft, either helicopter or airplane, these issues are further compounded by changes in altitude, which in turn affects humidity, atmospheric pressure, and oxygen concentration. Additional stress factors in air medical transportation include an even more confined patient care space; additional movement (up and down); and increased noise levels.

Multiple sedation scales have been widely used in the critical care setting but often lack significant testing for both validation and reliability [11,12]. Technology has evolved from the operating room and anesthesia that is currently being used in the critically ill patient to provide an objective measurement of sedation: the bispectral index monitor (Aspect Medical Systems, Newtown, Massachusetts). Although the bispectral index is being increasingly used in hospital settings [11,12], its use in the medical transportation setting is just being investigated [13]. A newer technology, actigraphy, has been studied in critically ill patients and compared favorably with standard sedation scales and other indices of sedation [12,14]. Although this technology holds great promise in the hospital setting, its use in the transport setting may be limited by its reliance on patient limb movement, which can certainly be caused by the movement and vibration of the vehicle. Further research is needed to determine if its use is feasible in the transportation arena.

Specialty patient types

Pediatric patients in a transport setting

Because most pediatric critical illnesses and injuries do not occur in proximity to a level 1 pediatric intensive care unit, there is the need for transportation to such facilities. The pediatric patient may be suffering from a variety of conditions that may require sedation. These conditions include respiratory distress requiring advanced airway management; head injuries secondary to accidental and nonaccidental trauma; pain related to trauma or medical conditions; and anxiety related to the injury, illness, or separation from their parents.

Providing sedation and comfort to ventilated children is an integral aspect of quality care. Appropriate sedation minimizes agitation, promotes ventilator synchrony, and helps relieve the anxiety and discomfort of the intensive care unit experience [15]. The same hypothesis holds when transporting a pediatric patient. The mainstay of sedation for the ventilated child is the concomitant use of opioids and benzodiazepines, both of which can be given in transport. Although opioids are analgesics, their use in combination with benzodiazepines provides synergistic sedation while also providing analgesia [16]. Both morphine and fentanyl are the most commonly used opioids in the ventilated pediatric patient. The benzodiazepines, such as midazolam and lorazepam, are both used for sedation. These two agents possess sedative, hypnotic, muscle relaxant, and anticonvulsant effects but no analgesia [16]. Propofol is a newer, very short-acting sedative-hypnotic agent that is used for short-term procedural sedation and for sedation of ventilated pediatric patients [16]. Propofol is a powerful sedative, characterized by rapid onset and short duration of action. Adverse effects include transient hypotension and dose-dependent respiratory depression [17]. Propofol controls stress responses and has anticonvulsant and amnesic properties [18]. It does not itself have analgesic properties but may be used in combination with opioids [18]. Although many of its actions are ideal for the transportation setting, there is little support in the literature for its use in this setting.

In the transportation setting, the nonventilated pediatric patient often needs sedation or pain management because of the type of injury they have suffered. Because the patient is not intubated, extra vigilance must be provided to detect potential adverse effects. In the case of fentanyl, an opiate 100 times more potent than morphine, the primary adverse effect is respiratory depression and resultant hyp-

oxia or apnea [19]. The primary adverse effects of midazolam are respiratory depression, paradoxical excitement, and occasional hypotension [19].

Maternal patients in a transport setting

There is a lack of information in the literature depicting the need or risk of sedation in the high-risk maternal patient during transportation. High-risk maternal patients are often transported from a smaller facility to a larger facility with level III neonatal intensive care unit capabilities. These patients are transferred because of the following reasons: premature rupture of membranes; premature labor; pregnancy-induced hypertension; and bleeding issues, such as abruption or placenta previa.

Pregnant women are also transported secondary to trauma. Of all injuries during pregnancy, 54% are from motor vehicle crashes; 70% of major, life-threatening injuries are from motor vehicle crashes [20]. Maternal mortality is most often caused by injuries sustained from motor vehicle crashes, specifically head injuries followed by multiple internal injuries [21]. Because protection of the airway is of utmost importance, the patient may need intubation [21]. Sedation is used as part of the RSI process.

Drugs administered to the pregnant woman during pregnancy can affect the fetus in a number of ways ranging from no effect to major structural or functional defects [22]. The fetus is a passive recipient of all drugs entering the mother's system. Medications are not "approved" for use in pregnancy; rather, medications are "presumed safe" for use in pregnancy [22].

Neonates in the transport setting

There is very little in the literature that addresses sedation of the critically ill neonate patient during a transport. There is much written about the sedation of the neonate in a hospital setting that also pertains to air or ground transportation.

The interfacility neonate transport patient is often a premature infant being moved from a small hospital to a level III neonatal intensive care unit with ventilator capabilities. The premature neonate usually requires intubation before transportation. If it is an emergent intubation, done shortly after the neonate is delivered, then sedation is not given because there is usually no venous access. If the neonate is nonemergently intubated before transportation, then sedation is given. Midazolam has been approved for use in neonates, and a randomized, controlled trial has demonstrated sedative effects. Adverse hemodynamic effects and abnormal movements have been associated with its use in the neonate; it is recommended that the dose be given either slowly by a continuous infusion, or by slow intravenous push [23].

Morphine is also used in the ventilated neonate for sedation. Morphine has been considered the gold standard of sedation in neonatal practice [24]. There are specific cases, such as meconium aspiration with persistent pulmonary hypertension, in which the use of nondepolarizing neuromuscular blocking agents and sedation enhance therapy. Nondepolarizing neuromuscular blocking agents and fentanyl are often the chosen combination in these cases [24].

Operational safety considerations

In addition to the usual considerations of patient care, the transportation setting adds an additional consideration of operational safety. With most ground and airplane transport vehicles, the patient is typically well isolated from the vehicle's operator by distance and physical barriers. In some types of helicopters, however, the patient is literally laying next to the pilot. Recognizing the potential threat to the safe operation of the vehicle, the Commission for Accreditation of Medical Transport Systems requires that each accredited program have a policy that addresses the use of both physical and chemical restraints for combative patients [25].

Complications

The medications typically used for sedation are not without adverse effects. Knowledge of those adverse effects and ability to treat them are an important aspect of their use [8]. Often these medications are used as a component of an RSI protocol. One study found a dose-related incidence of hypotension in prehospital patients subjected to an air medical transportation service RSI protocol using midazolam [26]. Green and Krauss [27] reviewed the use of propofol in the emergency room setting and identified that the most significant issue associated with its use was oversedation. They recommended the use of capnography and pulse oximetry for monitoring for hypoxia and hypoventilation. A group of physicians evaluated the incidence of adverse effects in relation to the use of sedation or analgesia in a prehospital setting for an entire year [28]. Although the study was based in France and used medications that are not available in the United States, their conclusions ring true for medical transport services everywhere. They recommended that measures include "…initial training, which must include training in the operating room and in intensive-care units, well known therapeutic protocols (including adapted doses of medication for frail patients), continuous training with daily monitoring of all medical reports concerning analgesia and anesthesia with discussion of side effect prevention…" [28].

Summary

Recognizing how the transportation setting affects the patient, and the required therapies to support the patient, is a critical aspect of patient care. Transporting an acutely or critically ill patient, be they neonatal, pediatric, maternal, adult medical, or trauma patients, requires an in-depth understanding of the application of sedation in the transportation setting, both therapeutic and adverse effects, and how to manage those effects for the best patient outcome.

References

[1] Stocking JC. Restraint and care within a confined space. In: Association of Air Medical Services (AAMS). Guidelines for air medical crew education. Dubuque (IA): Kendall/Hunt; 2004. p. 22-1-10.

[2] Klinker N. Air physiology. In: Association of Air Medical Services (AAMS). Guidelines for air medical crew education. Dubuque (IA): Kendall/Hunt; 2004. p. 14-1-11.

[3] Bolen R. Patient assessment and preparation. In: Association of Air Medical Services (AAMS). Guidelines for air medical crew education. Dubuque (IA): Kendall/Hunt; 2004. p. 15-1-21.

[4] Wilson D. Head, neck and facial trauma. In: Association of Air Medical Services (AAMS). Guidelines for air medical crew education. Dubuque (IA): Kendall/Hunt; 2004. p. 26-1-10.

[5] Carrubba C. Respiratory patients. In: Association of Air Medical Services (AAMS). Guidelines for air medical crew education. Dubuque (IA): Kendall/Hunt; 2004. p. 17-1-18.

[6] Emergency Nurses Association. Stabilization, transfer and transport. In: Jacobs BB, Hoyt KS, editors. Trauma nurse core curriculum. 4th edition. Des Plaines (IL): Emergency Nurses Association; 2000. p. 297-308.

[7] Adnet F, Lapostolle F, Ricard-Hibon A, et al. Intubating trauma patients before reaching hospital-revisited. Critical Care 2001;5:290-1.

[8] Allen MH, Currier GW, Hughes DH, et al. Expert Consensus Panel for Behavioral Emergencies. The

Expert Consensus Guideline Series. Treatment of behavioral emergencies. Postgrad Med 2001;(Spec No): 1–88.

[9] National Flight Nurses Association. Position statement: intravenous conscious sedation in air medical transport. Available at: www.astn.org/Position-papers/sedation.html. Accessed December 20, 2004.

[10] McMullan P, Carlton F, Summers RL, et al. The use of chemical restraint in helicopter transport. Air Med J 1999;18:136–9.

[11] Chulay M. Sedation assessment: easier said than done! Crit Care Nurs Clin N Am 2004;16:359–64.

[12] Lafleur KJ. Will adequate sedation assessment include the use of actigraphy in the future? Am J Crit Care 2005;14:61–3.

[13] Deschamp C, Carlton Jr FB, Phillips W, et al. The bispectral index monitor: a new tool for air medical personnel. Air Med J 2001;20:38–9.

[14] Grap MJ, Borchers CT, Munro CL, et al. Actigraphy in the critically ill: correlations with activity, agitation, and sedation. Am J Crit Care 2005;14:52–60.

[15] Brinker D. Sedation and comfort issues in the ventilated child and infant. Crit Care Nurs Clin N Am 2004;16:365–77.

[16] Brinker D. Pain management. In: Maloney-Harmon PA, Czerwinski SJ, editors. Nursing care of the pediatric trauma patient. St. Louis: WB Saunders; 2003. p. 118–37.

[17] Bassett KE, Anderson JL, Pribble CG, et al. Propofol for procedural sedation in children in the emergency department. Ann Emerg Med 2003;42:773–82.

[18] Guenther E, Pribble CG, Junkins Jr EP, et al. Propofol sedation by emergency physicians for elective pediatric outpatient procedures. Ann Emerg Med 2003;42: 783–91.

[19] American College of Emergency Physicians. Clinical policy: evidence-based approach to pharmacologic agents used in pediatric sedation and analgesia in the emergency department. Ann Emerg Med 2004;44: 342–77.

[20] Gilbert ES, Harmon JS. Trauma. In: Manual of high risk pregnancy and delivery. 3rd edition. St. Louis: Mosby; 2003. p. 534–48.

[21] Daddario J. Trauma in pregnancy. In: Manderville LK, Troiano NH, editors. High-risk and critical care intrapartum nursing. 2nd edition. Philadelphia: Lippincott; 1999. p. 322–52.

[22] Blackburn ST. Pharmacology and pharmacokinetics during the perinatal period. In: Ledbetter MS, editor. Maternal, fetal and neonatal physiology: a clinical perspective. 2nd edition. St. Louis: WB Saunders; 2003. p. 180–212.

[23] American Academy of Pediatrics. Policy statement: prevention and management of pain and stress in the neonate. Pediatrics 2000;105:454–61.

[24] Aoki BY, McCloskey K. Neonatal emergencies. In: Manning S, editor. Evaluation, stabilization, and transport of the critically ill child. St. Louis: Mosby; 1992. p. 307–19.

[25] Commission on Accreditation of Medical Transport Systems. Accreditation standards of the commission on accreditation of medical transport systems. 6th edition. Anderson (SC): Commission on Accreditation of Medical Transport Systems; 2004.

[26] Davis DP, Kimbro TA, Vilke GM. The use of midazolam for prehospital rapid-sequence intubation may be associated with a dose-related increase in hypotension. Prehosp Emerg Care 2001;5:163–8.

[27] Green SM, Krauss B. Propofol in emergency medicine: pushing the sedation frontier. Ann Emerg Med 2003; 42:792–7.

[28] Ricard-Hibon A, Chollet C, Belpomme V, et al. Epidemiology of adverse effects of prehospital sedation analgesia. Am J Emerg Med 2003;21:461–6.

ELSEVIER
SAUNDERS

CRITICAL CARE
NURSING CLINICS
OF NORTH AMERICA

Crit Care Nurs Clin N Am 17 (2005) 211 – 223

Tolerance and Withdrawal Issues with Sedation

Antonia Zapantis, MS, PharmD[a,b,*], Simon Leung, PharmD[a,c]

[a]Department of Pharmacy Practice, College of Pharmacy, Nova Southeastern University, 3200 South University Drive,
Fort Lauderdale, FL 33328, USA
[b]Department of Pharmacy, North Broward Medical Center, 201 East Sample Road, Deerfield Beach, FL 33064, USA
[c]Department of Pharmacy, Cleveland Clinic Hospital, 3100 Weston Road, Weston, FL 33331, USA

The stay in an ICU is a complex mixture of providing optimal care while keeping the patient safe. Critically ill patients are often agitated and anxious. Means of reducing the anxiety associated with the ICU stay include frequent reorientation and maintenance of patient comfort with sedation supplemented by analgesia as needed. Sedation may also help facilitate mechanical ventilation [1]. Various agents are used to provide sedation. The most common include benzodiazepines (BZDs), propofol, and the newer dexmedetomidine (DEX). Others include barbiturate agents (thiopental and pentobarbital); neuroleptics (chlorpromazine, droperidol, haloperidol); clonidine; etomidate; ketamine; and supplemental opioid analgesics for pain control.

A common complication of sedation, especially in patients sedated for more than 1 week, is tolerance, which can lead to withdrawal if the sedation is discontinued hastily [1]. This article evaluates the occurrence of tolerance and withdrawal in the most commonly used sedatives in critically ill patients.

Tolerance is defined as a progressive reduction in drug effect when a constant dose is given over a period of time [2,3]. Increased doses are required to achieve the effects originally produced by lower doses. It is a pharmacologic effect from physiologic changes that induce a progressive loss of sensitivity to the drug [4]. Tolerance in this setting can present as metabolic or functional. By increasing the rate of

metabolism of the substance, the body may be able to eliminate the substance more readily [3,5]. Functional tolerance is a decrease in sensitivity of the central nervous system (CNS) to the substance [3]. Receptor site tolerance is a decrease in the drug effect with repeated doses despite the drug accumulation within the body. An easily recognizable example of tolerance in the outpatient setting is a decrease in the level of drowsiness after the first few days of oral BZD therapy [5]. Cross-tolerance is a situation when the nervous system becomes tolerant to one drug and then adapts in a similar way to a different drug more rapidly [2].

Withdrawal syndrome is a group of symptoms that occur with the cessation or reduction of use of a psychoactive substance that has been taken repeatedly, usually for a prolonged period or in high doses [3]. The manifestations of withdrawal vary according to the agent used for sedation, manifesting shortly after discontinuation of the drug if the agent has a short half-life (propofol, fentanyl) or days later if the agent or its metabolites have long half-lives (diazepam). Delayed clearance of active metabolites or the parent compound in patients with underlying renal or hepatic dysfunction may also delay the onset of the withdrawal symptoms [6]. The onset and course of withdrawal are time-limited and are related to the type of substance and dose being taken immediately before cessation or dose reduction. Typically, the features of withdrawal are the opposite of those of acute intoxication. Sedative withdrawal syndromes have many features in common with alcohol withdrawal (tremor, sweating, anxiety, agitation, depression, nausea, and malaise), but may also include muscle aches and twitches, perceptual distortions,

---

* Corresponding author. College of Pharmacy, Nova Southeastern University, 3200 South University Drive, Fort Lauderdale, FL 33328.

E-mail address: zapantis@nsu.nova.edu (A. Zapantis).

0899-5885/05/$ – see front matter © 2005 Elsevier Inc. All rights reserved.
doi:10.1016/j.ccell.2005.04.011

and distortions of body image. Opioid withdrawal is accompanied by rhinorrhea (running nose); lacrimation (excessive tear formation); aching muscles; chills; gooseflesh; and, after 24 to 48 hours, muscle and abdominal cramps [3]. Dependence has referred to physical manifestations of withdrawal resulting from the body's physiologic adaptation to long-term drug use [4]. Such withdrawal has been described following seemingly brief use (greater than 48 hours) and is much more common if the agent is discontinued abruptly [2]. Withdrawal is a diagnosis of exclusion and in the pediatric population fever or vomiting should never be attributed to withdrawal until other possible causes are excluded [6]. Administration of high doses of BZDs increases the risk of developing moderate-to-severe withdrawal reactions. The concurrent administration of cross-dependent drugs (eg, barbiturates) increases the occurrence of withdrawal reactions [7]. The American College of Critical Care Medicine recommends that the potential for opioid, BZD, and propofol withdrawal should be considered after high doses or more than approximately 7 days of continuous therapy. Doses should be tapered systematically to prevent withdrawal symptoms [1].

This complication is a known problem in sedation. In a survey of critical care fellows, most (61.8%) reported seeing withdrawal in their institution after discontinuation of sedation and that treatment was instituted after identification of withdrawal symptoms. Only 23.5% of the centers, however, routinely tapered (range 2 days–6 weeks) sedative dosages to prevent withdrawal [8]. Of note, withdrawal symptoms are rarely noted postoperatively, possibly because analgesia is weaned over several days as pain lessens [2]. The critical care nurse plays a pivotal role in ensuring that adequate sedation and analgesia are achieved and critically ill patients do not experience untoward effects. Furthermore, in collaboration with medical staff, they should ensure that patients are properly weaned from sedatives and analgesics so that withdrawal symptoms are avoided [4].

In addition to tolerance and withdrawal issues, critically ill patients have altered sedative and analgesic pharmacokinetics and pharmacodynamics. The altered pharmacokinetic properties manifest as a variety of problems. These drugs are generally highly protein bound and primarily eliminated by the liver, making them susceptible to a variety of drug interactions. Drug elimination is generally impaired in the critically ill. Hypoperfusion of liver and renal tissues slow drug delivery to these organs and may reduce excretion. Most sedatives and analgesics used

for long periods of time are prone to accumulation, resulting in prolonged drug effects. In addition to altered pharmacokinetic properties, these drugs also have altered pharmacodynamic properties. Metabolic disturbances along with organ dysfunction can diminish drug efficacy or increase risk of toxicity. These issues are further complicated in the neonatal population [9]. This population has delayed drug elimination as compared with adults with a large pharmacokinetic interindividual variability [10]. Knowledge of sedative and analgesic pharmacology and application of continuous clinical monitoring are essential to the delivery of appropriate and cost-effective pharmaceutical care to the critically ill patient [9].

Benzodiazepines

To fully understand the mechanism of action of BZD tolerance and withdrawal, it is important to be knowledgeable of BZD pharmacology. BZDs exert their actions by attaching to the γ-aminobutyric acid receptor on cells in the CNS reducing cellular excitability [2]. This inhibition promotes sedation [4]. Chronic BZD administration results in downregulation of these receptors, which leads to decreased pharmacologic efficacy resulting in less inhibition of the CNS (ie, tolerance occurs) [6]. More BZD is needed to achieve the same effect [4].

Robb and Hargrave [5] found that patients with history of oral BZD showed tolerance to the sedative and respiratory depressant effects of midazolam when it was administered for dental procedures. Other studies have found that tolerance can occur even during short-term administration of BZDs. Coldwell and coworkers [11] found during acute administration of midazolam motor control task performance improved, even though plasma concentrations increased slightly. They concluded that subjects developed acute tolerance to the effects of midazolam within the 70-minute infusion period. In another similar study, the researchers found that performance improved even while alprazolam concentrations were held constant during the short-term (<36 hours) continuous infusion [12]. Others have found that toward end of the studied intubation period, unusually large amounts of midazolam were required to achieve optimal sedation, implying midazolam resistance [13]. It has also been suggested that tolerance develops more rapidly with the continuous versus intermittent administration of sedative and analgesic agents [6]. Cross-tolerance is also associated with chronic use of alcohol. Doses of BZDs to produce adequate sedation need to be higher than normally used in patients who regularly use BZDs or who drank large amounts of alcohol. Blood levels required to produce sedation need to be dramatically increased [5]. Although in this population physical dependency and withdrawal is considered to be a result of what has been administered in the ICU, it may also result from medications that the patient received before admission. This is why it is even more important to consider outpatient medication and social history when initiating sedatives. Proper dose titration from the manufacturer-recommended dosages is necessary to provide the desired level of sedation [6]. Conversely, high doses of BZDs are needed to overcome any tolerance developed to achieve sedation during acute BZD or alcohol withdrawal [4,14].

Withdrawal of BZDs from critical care patients may produce an abstinence syndrome, including increasing anxiety, fear, dread, and confusion and agitation with abrupt withdrawal, increasing patients' risk for refractory seizures [4]. A retrospective chart review of over 27,000 patients evaluated the incidence of new-onset seizures in the medical or surgical ICU during an 11-year period. Fifty-five patients (58% women) with an age range of 31 to 87 years old were identified with new-onset seizures. Of those, 18 patients had sudden drug withdrawal (17 narcotics and 1 midazolam). The one patient with midazolam withdrawal had 12 days of therapy. All seizures occurred within 2 to 4 days after sudden withdrawal and were generalized tonic-clonic seizures [15].

Many cases of BZD withdrawal have been described in the literature. Table 1 describes 16 cases, mostly pediatric, of BZD withdrawal. The 14 pediatric cases (age 14 days to 15 years old) were mostly female (N = 8). The primary diagnosis for these patients included surgery; skull fracture; burn; infections (bronchiolitis, respiratory syncytial virus infection, septicemia, pneumonia); asthma; congestive heart failure; seizures; and metastatic disease. The average midazolam dose ranged from 2.4 to 24 µg/kg/min with one midazolam withdrawal episode treated with clorazepate, 2 mg/h orally. Duration of sedation ranged from 11 hours to 2 months. Sedation was weaned over 6 hours to 4 days, but most were described merely as "abruptly." Withdrawal symptoms appeared within 12 to 24 hours after the infusion rate was decreased or discontinued. Withdrawal symptoms seen included jitteriness, irritability, agitation, fussiness, grimacing, hyperactivity, aggression, uncommunicative, inconsolable or high pitch crying, poor feeding, gagging, vomiting, tachycardia, abnormal movement, tremors, sleeplessness, poor social interaction, inability for eyes to fix or follow movement, inability to locate noxious stimulus, hallucinations, and in one case two episodes of general convulsions. Most patients were restarted on the sedation and weaning was reinitiated usually at a slower dose [13,16–19]. The two adult cases included in Table 1 were one woman patient (36 years old) and one man patient (53 years old). The first case was admitted to the ICU for a tricyclic antidepressant overdose with no seizure activity. The patient was sedated with a total dose of 13,440 mg of midazolam over 33 days (407 mg average daily dose), which was discontinued within two days. Within six hours this resulted in anxiety, agitation, EEG identified seizures, and loss of consciousness. The symptoms were treated acutely with clonazepam 1 mg, then reinitiating midazolam at 10 mg/hr, clonazepam continuously infused at a daily dose of 3 mg, and chlorazepate as needed for insomnia [20]. The second adult case was given midazolam in intermittent doses (22 mg average daily dose) for 21 days, which was abruptly discontinued. Within five hours this resulted in severe diffuse arthralgias and myalgias, tachycardia, fever, and increased anxiety. The symptoms were treated with a bolus of midazolam and reinitiating previous schedule, which was then tapered over four days successfully [21].

A number of retrospective chart reviews have also evaluated the incidence of withdrawal after discontinuation of BZDs in both pediatric and adult populations. In the three studies evaluating the incidence of BZD withdrawal in children, the patients were receiving concurrent analgesia. Fonsmark and coworkers [7] conducted a retrospective chart review of 40 children 6 months to 14 years of age with midazolam being the primary sedative used. If adequate sedation was not achieved, pentobarbital was added to therapy or replaced midazolam. All patients received analgesia with morphine. Symptoms were classified as mild or severe. Mild symptoms included anxiety, insomnia, restlessness, and tremor. Severe symptoms included confusion, psychosis, and seizures. Of these patients, 35% experienced withdrawal symptoms. Eight were sedated with both midazolam and pentobarbital, three received only midazolam, and three received only pentobarbital. The researchers believed that the patients on both midazolam and pentobarbital might have developed tolerance. Length of stay, duration of sedation, and duration of mechanical ventilation were significantly longer in children exhibiting withdrawal symptoms. Classic opiate withdrawal syndrome (yawning, sneezing, lacrimation, gooseflesh) was not observed implicating the withdrawal symptoms to be from either the BZD or pentobarbital. Patients being treated with

Table 1
Reports of BDZ withdrawal syndrome

Patient type	Sex	Age	Mean midazolam dose (μg/kg/min)	Comorbidities	Symptoms
Peds	M	14 d	1st infusion: 4.75	Cardiac surgery	Restlessness, bulging stomach, V
			2nd infusion: 2.4, then weaned to 0.6. Chlorazepate 2 mg/h PO started to prevent WD from midazolam		Restlessness, bulging stomach, tachycardia, V
Peds	M	2 m	5	Bronchiolitis	IC, moving all limbs, sleeplessness, PF
Peds	F	3 m	ND	CHF, mitral regurgitation, RSV infection, cardiac surgery	Child did not smile, coo, or grasp; unusual movements of tongue and ext; dyskinetic movements of the mouth; stiff posture
Peds	F	5 m	1st infusion: 24 (inadvertantly)	Bronchiolitis	Gagging, V
			2nd infusion: 5		Jitteriness, gagging, V, PF
Peds	F	5 m	ND	RSV pneumonia	Poor social interaction, irritability, high-pitched cry, arching of back, stiff/abnormal movements, inability to swallow
Peds	M	7 m	4	Skull fracture	IC, V, coughing, tachycardia
Peds	F	11 m	5	Surgical repair of tetralogy of Fallot	IC, jitteriness, PF
Peds	M	15 m	1st infusion: 3.6	SZ, apneic episodes, septicemia	Restlessness, tachycardia, V
			2nd infusion: 2.4		
Peds	F	15 m	ND	Down syndrome, asthma, cardiac surgery, cardiac arrest during surgery	Poor social interaction, eyes did not fix or follow movement, could not locate noxious stimulus
Peds	F	16 m	5	Burn	IC, irritability, agitation, fussiness, grimacing
Peds	M	4 y	3.7	Pneumonia	Hyperactive, aggressive, uncommunicative, visual hallucinations, did not recognize parents
Peds	F	11 y	2.8	Acute severe asthmatic attack	Visual hallucinations and two episodes general convulsions
Peds	F	12 y	9.3	Acute severe asthmatic attack	Agitation, uncommunicative, abusive, repetitive facial grimacing
Peds	M	15 y	ND	Metastatic disease	Tremors, hallucinations, with intensification over the next 48 h
Adult	F	36 y	Total dose = 13,440 mg; average daily dose = 407 mg; average hourly does = 17 mg/h	TCA overdose with no seizure activity	Anxiety, agitation, SZ identified on EEG, loss of consciousness
Adult	M	53 y	Intermittent doses; average daily dose = 22 mg	Rheumatoid arthritis, GI obstruction and surgery, pneumonia, pseudomonal sepsis	Severe, diffuse arthralgias and myalgias, tachycardia, febrile, increasingly anxious and demanding

Abbreviations: CHF, congestive heart failure; EEG; electroencephalogram; F, female; GI, gastrointestinal; IC, inconsolable crying; IVP, intravenous push; M, male; ND, no data; NMB, neuromuscular blocker; PF, poor feeding; PO, oral; RSV, respiratory syncytial virus; SZ, seizure; V, vomiting; WD, withdraw.

Duration of sedation	Duration of weaning	Time symptoms occur after weaning of infusion	Outcome	Ref
29 d	ND	12 h	Midazolam infusion restarted at 2.4 μg/kg/min. All symptoms disappeared	[18]
2 m	Chlorazepate was discontinued abruptly	12 h	Chlorazepate 285 μg/kg/h by continuous infusion. All symptoms disappeared.	
6 d with fentanyl	6 h	Within 12 h	ND	[16]
5 d concurrently with fentanyl	ND	ND	2 wk after neurologic examination	[17]
11 h	4 d	Within 12 h	Restarted midazolam at 5 μg/kg/min	[16]
4 d	36 h	Within 24 h	ND	
5 d with fentanyl	ND	ND	Gradual improvement and 5 wk later, neurologic examination returned to normal	[17]
9 d with fentanyl	2.5 d	Within 13 h	ND	[16]
3 d with fentanyl	10 h	Within 24 h	ND	[16]
12 d	ND	12 h	Midazolam infusion restarted at 2.4 μg/kg/min. All symptoms disappeared	[18]
4 d	ND	12 h	Midazolam infusion restarted at 4.7 μg/kg/min. All symptoms disappeared. After 1 wk because of inadequate sedation rate increased to 9.5 μg/kg/min. Then switched to clorazepate at 0.85 μg/kg/min and weaned successfully after 2 wk	
10 d with fentanyl and NMB	ND	ND	6 weeks normal except patient could not crawl or grasp as she had done prior to admission. After 5 mo she was crawling and grasping normally.	[17]
16 d with morphine	4 d	Within 12 h	ND	[16]
7 d with NMB	ND	24 h	Chlorpromazine and chloral hydrate provided temporary sedation, but only diazepam (IV and PO) provided partial relief of symptoms. Diazepam continued for 7 d until behavior returned to normal	[13]
14 d with NMB	ND	24 h	Treated with IV diazepam, then oral diazepam to treat a confusional state for 2 d	[13]
17 d with morphine & NMB	ND	24 h	Treated with diazepam IV for 24 h to suppress abnormal behavior	[13]
33 d with fentanyl	ND	Soon	Morphine and diazepam did not control symptoms; midazolam infusion was restarted	[19]
33 d	2 d	6 h	Acutely treated with clonazepam 1 mg, then restart midazolam at 10 mg/h, clonazepam continuously infused at daily dose of 3 mg, chlorazepate for insomnia	[20]
21 d	Abruptly	5 h	Treated with midazolam 2 mg IVP (9 h after last dose). Resumed previous midazolam schedule. Tapered over 4 d successfully. Patient expired 2 mo later because of sepsis complications	[21]

higher total doses of midazolam ($\geq$60 mg/kg) or pentobarbital ($\geq$25 mg/kg) were more likely to experience withdrawal symptoms ($P < .05$).

Bergmen et al [17] conducted a chart review of all pediatric patients who had received continuous midazolam infusions during an unspecified period of time and identified five female patients exhibiting neurologic abnormalities. Three of these cases were described comprehensively and are included in Table 1. The average age of the children was 3.94 years (range 0.03–19.2). Primary diagnoses of the patients included respiratory syncytial virus bronchiolitis, Down syndrome, asthma, history of cardiac surgery, coronary artery repair, and atrial and ventricular septal defects. The average total midazolam dose was 29.8 mg/kg (range 1.4–286) with an average duration of 128 hours (range 12–917). All patients also received fentanyl and the average total dose was 179 μg/kg (range 1–2934). Duration of weaning and onset of withdrawal symptoms were not provided. Symptoms included decreased responsiveness, tongue thrusting, staring, and shaking. Patients with definite and possible neurologic sequelae from sedation were associated with young age ($P = .025$); female gender ($P = .017$); low serum albumin ($P = .036$); and concomitant aminophylline administration ($P = .037$). The neurologic abnormalities persisted for 5 days to 4 weeks but completely resolved in all cases [6].

In a prospectively repeated measures study design, the occurrence and severity of withdrawal symptoms were described. The symptoms were identified using a standardized assessment tool and clinical management guidelines. During an 11-month period, 15 children (age 6 weeks–28 months) met the inclusion criteria of at least 4 days of opioid and BZD therapy with withdrawal symptoms after initiation of weaning. Fourteen of the patients underwent cardiac surgery for various diagnoses and five of these children required extracorporeal membrane oxygenation following failure to wean from bypass. One patient was being medically treated only for cardiac failure. Thirteen patients received both opioid and midazolam, whereas two children received opioids alone. Most of the children received at least one other drug during the weaning period, such as chloral hydrate (N = 10); clonidine (N = 9); or lorazepam (N = 3). The median cumulative midazolam dose was 29.8 mg/kg (range 1.4–286) with a peak of 4 μg/kg/min (range 0–13.6). The median cumulative opioid dose was 7.36 mg/kg (range 2.48–19.2) during 9-day duration (range 4–18 days) with a peak of 40 μg/kg/min (range 20–131). The children who received extracorporeal membrane oxygenation ther-

apy required larger cumulative and peak doses of opioids. The onset of symptoms occurred 2 days (range 0–6) after the taper began and moderate to severe withdrawal symptoms lasted 3 days (range 0–12). Shorter duration of tapering and higher dose correlated with withdrawal symptoms [22].

In a chart review, adult burn patients with inhalation injury receiving mechanical ventilation with continuous infusions of BZDs and opioids were evaluated to determine the incidence of withdrawal syndrome. Eleven patients (age 37 ± 3 years) out of 324 reviewed with lorazepam or midazolam use for greater than 7 days were identified to have mild to severe signs and symptoms of withdrawal. Most of the patients were men (N = 8). Symptoms included confusion, diaphoresis, muscle twitching, picking motion, and seizures. Most of the symptoms were mild and did not influence the rate of weaning. Of note, two patients did experience BZD withdrawal seizures. Number and severity of withdrawal symptoms were related to rate of drug weaning in both opioids and BZDs and were not related to peak dose, total dose, or duration before weaning phase [23].

Cammarano and coworkers [24] reviewed the incidence of withdrawal symptoms in adult mechanically ventilated ICU patients. Twenty-eight patients met the inclusion criteria and of those, nine met criteria for a diagnosis of acute withdrawal syndrome. Signs and symptoms of BZD withdrawal included dysphoria, tremor, headache, nausea, sweating, fatigue, anxiety, agitation, increased sensitivity to light and sound, paresthesias, strange sensations, muscle cramps, myoclonus, sleep disturbances, dizziness, delirium, and seizure. This review showed that patients exhibiting withdrawal were younger (34.9 ± 4.6 versus 50.9 ± 4 years, $P = .017$) and were more likely to have acute respiratory distress syndrome with seven (77.8%) of nine patients experiencing withdrawal versus 5 (26.3%) of 19 patients with no withdrawal symptoms. Patients experiencing withdrawal were more likely to have greater than 1 day concurrent propofol ($P = .013$) or neuromuscular blockade ($P = .004$). Sedative and narcotic titration is more difficult in patients receiving concomitant neuromuscular blockade because neuromuscular blockade suppresses the usual clues for assessment of sedation or pain. Also, these patients receive higher doses of sedatives and analgesics to avoid undetected awareness and pain. There was no difference in specific opioid or BZD administered. In addition, patients manifesting withdrawal had longer periods of mechanical ventilation (39.6 ± 7.1 versus 21.3 ± 4.8 days, $P = .049$); BZD duration (38.2 ± 7.5 versus 19.6 ± 4 days, $P = .049$); and propofol duration

(18.6 ± 5 versus 6.6 ± 1.9, $P = .049$). This could possibly be explained by the fact that acute respiratory distress syndrome typically increases mechanical ventilation duration. They had significantly higher mean daily doses of narcotic (6.4 ± 2.1 versus 1.4 ± 0.2 mg) and lorazepam equivalent dose (37.8 ± 11.8 versus 11.1 ± 3.2 mg). Because tolerance can occur within days and in this study BZD mean duration was longer than the time required to develop tolerance and increased dose requirements, tolerance was likely. Also, although it was not statistically significant, withdrawal patients were weaned two times faster than nonwithdrawal patients. Extended ICU care (≥7 days) and larger sedative doses increase the risk for acute withdrawal syndromes during drug weaning [24].

Propofol

Structurally unrelated to BZDs, propofol (2,6-diisopropylphenol) is a phenol derivative that exhibits sedative-hypnotic activity [25,26]. Propofol is considered an ideal sedative because of its rapid onset of action, short duration of effect, easy titration, rapid dissipation of effect, limited accumulation, minimal side effects, and absence of active metabolites. The exact mechanism of action of propofol is not entirely certain. It is postulated, however, that the CNS depressive effects are caused by the activation of γ-aminobutyric acid receptors in the CNS, similar to the action of BZDs [27]. The incidence of tolerance to propofol is unpredictable and the mechanisms to the development of tolerance are thought to be complex and multifactorial. Pharmacokinetic tolerance, which results from a change in the absorption, distribution, metabolism, or excretion of a drug that effectively reduces the concentration of the drug at its receptors, produces no more than a threefold decrease in response to the drug. Pharmacodynamic tolerance results from adaptive changes within the organism so that the response to a given concentration of drug is reduced. This typically involves changes in the availability of drug receptor or receptor responsiveness (up- or down-regulation), and the magnitude of tolerance can vary.

Since the introduction of propofol in the market, there are three publications of tolerance to propofol reported in adult ICU patients (Table 2) [28–30]. A small European pilot study conducted on mechanically ventilated patients (N = 11) demonstrated that 27% of patients who received propofol concurrently with alfentanil for more than 5 days developed tolerance, which was defined as an increased infusion rate with an accompanying increase in blood concentration at a constant Ramsay Score of 3 [28]. Nevertheless, the author suggested that extrahepatic clearance, increased volume of distribution in certain diseases, and severity of illness might contribute to the development of tolerance. In addition, two small European studies (N = 22 and N = 9) suggested that the development of tolerance tended to occur after 7 days of continuous propofol infusion [29,30]. It is difficult to extrapolate information from these studies because of the lack of detailed description of the methodology and the variability among study subjects and environments. It has been documented that the total body clearances of propofol (91–156 L per hour)

Table 2
Reports of propofol tolerance after continuous infusion

Pt type	No. of Pts	Age (y)	Diagnosis	Bolus (mg/kg)	MD (mg/kg/h)	Concomitant analgesic	% of pts developed tolerance	Duration of sedation	Ref.
Adult ICU	11	56.9 ± 17.7	ARDS, RF, RI, O	ND	ND	Alfentanil	27	5–10 d	[28]
Adult ICU	22	19 – 76	ND	0.03–0.8	0.6–13.8	ND	—	0.5–14 d	[29]
Adult ICU	9	ND	ND	ND	ND	Alfentanil or morphine	ND	7–30 d	[30]
Peds OP	10	2.7 ± 1	Rad therapy	ND	30 ± 21	Ketamine or midazolam	0	13 ± 9 min, 134 Tx	[32]
Peds OP	6	2.0 ± 1.2	Rad therapy	initially 1, then 0.5	6–30	ND	0	27 ± 8 Tx	[33]
Peds OP	1	2	Rad therapy	1–18	0.1–0.5	None	100	15 min, 23 Tx	[34]
Peds OP	15	2.5 – 10	Rad therapy	5	9	None	0	24 ± 5 Tx	[35]
Peds OP	2	ND	Rad therapy	ND	ND	ND	0	>50 Tx	[36]

Abbreviations: ARDS, acute respiratory distress syndrome; ND, no data; O, others; OP, outpatient; Pt, patient; Rad, radiation; RF, respiratory failure; RI, respiratory infection; Tx, treatment.

Table 3
Reports of propofol withdrawal syndrome

Age	Sex	Dose (μg/kg/min)	Diagnosed injury	Comorbidities	Symptoms	Duration of sedation	Duration of weaning	Time of symptoms occur after weaning of infusion	Outcome	Ref
48 y	M	5–35	Thermal, 30% TBSA	EtOH abuse, bipolar	Agitation, tremors, tachycardia, tachypnea, hyperpyrexia	>83 d	4 and 2 d	6 and 39 h	Death	[27]
22 y	F	50–200	Sepsis	—	Tonic-clonic SZ	13 d	ND	6 d	Survived	[37]
41 y	F	ND	Aortic dissection	None	Confusion, tremors, hallucinations, grand-mal SZ	5 d	ND	0–10 h	Survived	[38]
31 y	M	initial 2.5 mg/kg, intermittent boluses total 5 mg/kg	Vasectomy	None	Tonic-clonic SZ	ND	ND	0.5 h	Survived	[39]
18 m	F	ND	Thermal, 20% TBSA	ND	Generalized twitching	14 d	ND	ND	Unknown	[40]

Abbreviations: EtOH, alcohol; F, female; M, male; ND, no data; SZ, seizure; TBSA, total body surface area.

in both short- and long-term infusions for anesthesia exceed normal hepatic blood flow suggesting the possibility of pulmonary clearance [26]. Furthermore, cross-tolerance has not been reported in humans with propofol and other sedative-hypnotic agents and other analgesics. This may be explained by propofol's unique structure and pharmacologic properties, suggesting a separate receptor-binding site to induce the sedative-hypnotic effect. In the case of propofol tolerance, it is recommended that either the infusion be discontinued or the rate be decreased and another sedative added to achieve the desired sedation levels [25]. The lipid profile, particularly triglycerides, should also be monitored closely if infusion continues beyond 48 hours or infusion rates escalate because of apparent tolerance, because this can lead to elevated triglyceride levels [1].

Although the manufacturer does not recommend propofol use in pediatric ICU patients because of its increased mortality rate, it continues to be used in pediatric anesthesia outside of the ICU arena [31]. Conflicting clinical data have been reported on the development of increased tolerance to propofol after repeated exposures over time for deep sedation or general anesthesia in small children with malignancies requiring high-voltage outpatient radiation therapy (see Table 2) [32–36]. Caution should be exercised in interpreting these data, however, because of flaws of study design, small sample size, and variability among patients and their disease states. Until larger and well-controlled studies are conducted to confirm the safety of propofol use in the pediatric population, the use of this agent in an outpatient setting should continue to be under extreme caution.

Although propofol is considered as safe and well tolerated in adults when used in short-term sedation (less than 72 hours), long-term administration of propofol has been associated with withdrawal syndrome that occurs with dosage reduction or an abrupt discontinuation of propofol continuous infusion in the critical care settings. There have been five cases of adverse events associated with withdrawal syndrome after propofol infusion (Table 3) [27,37–40]. Cawley and coworkers [27] described a severely burned, mechanically ventilated, septic patient who received propofol for sedation caused by difficulty in maintaining adequate sedation from lorazepam and morphine, and experienced withdrawal syndrome during weaning from propofol. On two separate occasions (108 and 113 days of hospital stay), 6 and 39 hours after weaning off propofol, the patient experienced sudden symptoms of agitation, tremor, tachycardia, tachypnea, and hyperpyrexia. Both incidents were resolved by reinitiating propofol infusion

at 5 μg/kg/min [27]. In adults, three reports have been documented of seizure activity 5 or 6 days after discontinuation of propofol infusion [37–39]. This phenomenon may be related to propofol's conflicting anticonvulsant and neuroexcitatory activities, which require further investigation [26,41,42]. It was noted that the dose of propofol used in one of these patients was higher than other published cases [37]. One report described a pediatric (18 month old) burn patient sedated and mechanically ventilated for 14 days who experienced generalized twitching after terminating the infusion [40]. An infusion lasting more than 5 days may increase the risk of withdrawal syndrome. Age, gender, dose, comorbidity, and duration of weaning do not seem, however, to play a major role in the emergence of propofol withdrawal syndrome.

Dexmedetomidine

DEX, an imidazole derivative, is a highly selective α_2-adrenergic receptor agonist with eight times higher affinity to the α2-adrenergic receptor than clonidine [43,44]. DEX administered as a continuous infusion of less than 24 hours is indicated for sedation of initially intubated and mechanically ventilated patients during treatment in the ICU settings [45]. The sedative-hypnotic effect of DEX is mediated through postsynaptic α_2-adrenergic receptors, which are coupled to pertussis toxin-sensitive G_i proteins in the CNS. Once activated, these G_i-proteins allow opening of the potassium channels and efflux of potassium ions causing hyperpolarization of the neuronal cell. This phenomenon leads to a reduction in firing of excitable cells in the CNS. Other effects of DEX include a decrease in calcium-ion conductance through N-type voltage-gated transmembrane calcium channels leading to inhibition of neurotransmitter release. The diversity of pharmacologic effects of DEX may also include stimulation of phospholipase A_2 activity, increased Na^+/H^+ exchange, and elevated polyphosphoinositide hydrolysis through α_2-adrenergic receptor activation [46,47].

Tolerance to DEX in humans has not been reported. Similar to clonidine, however, a partial α_2-adrenergic receptor agonist, this phenomenon has been documented extensively in a number of animal studies [48–52]. Although the precise mechanism for the development of tolerance to DEX has not been fully elucidated, it is thought to involve receptor desensitization through a loss of receptors or receptor-effector uncoupling [53]. Tolerance to the hypnotic effect develops in chronic administration, approximately 7 days in rats, with a more pronounced effect after 14 days [50–52]. This response disappears when the drug is discontinued. Tolerance to the analgesic effect of DEX occurs less frequently in rats compared with clonidine after chronic administration [52]. Furthermore, tolerance does not develop for either the sympatholytic (blunting of sympathetic activities) or minimum halothane anesthetic concentration sparing effect of DEX in rats [54]. Using electroencephalogram to measure the hypnotic effect of DEX in rats, tolerance does not appear in increased infusion rate of DEX ranging from 0.1 to 2 μg/kg/min over a total duration of up to 4 days [55], although other animal studies suggest more than 7 days is needed for tolerance to develop [50–52]. In animal models, hypnotic tolerance develops sooner than analgesic tolerance, whereas sympatholytic tolerance is unlikely to occur.

Cross-tolerance between DEX and other BZDs has not been reported in the literature. Animal studies have suggested, however, that cross-tolerance between DEX and clonidine is unlikely to occur [52]. Further studies are needed to confirm these findings in humans. This observation has also been demonstrated between DEX and morphine in animal models suggesting a functional linkage between the *mu* opioid and α_2-adrenergic receptors [56,57]. In morphine-tolerant rats, the development of cross-tolerance to the hypnotic effects of DEX appears after 4 days, whereas cross-tolerance to the analgesic properties of DEX requires a longer period of time [55]. This can be explained by a comparatively larger receptor reserve for the analgesic response in the spinal cord than for those needed for the hypnotic response [50–52]. It is difficult to extrapolate these data for humans because there are a number of limitations in these animal studies and the results have not been confirmed in clinical studies, although there is a potential for cross-tolerance.

Anecdotal data suggest DEX may play a role in facilitating opioid and BZD withdrawal in critically ill adult and pediatric patients. When DEX was gradually tapered over 36 hours to 7 days, signs and symptoms of withdrawal were not observed [58–60]. Rebound effects on the hemodynamics and behavior and other withdrawal symptoms after cessation of chronic DEX infusion have yet to be determined. Hyperalgesia has been described as one of the phenomena of opioid withdrawal after chronic administration in humans and animal models and this observation can be associated with decreased opioid levels from inadvertent or purposeful termination of opioids [61–64]. In humans, it is not known whether hyperalgesia occurs as DEX serum levels decline.

In animal models, however, hyperalgesia (up to 72 hours) does not occur after cessation of relative long-term (5 days) DEX administration [65].

Withdrawal strategies

When discontinuing sedatives following prolonged use, tapering should occur over several days [66]. Smaller doses are given and there is a reduced risk of tolerance with the use of sedation scales that facilitate appropriate titration [6]. Every effort should be made to prevent withdrawal symptoms [2]. Weaning can be done rapidly (10%–15% every 6–8 hours) in patients with short-term use (< 3–5 days). After prolonged administration, however, weaning may take 2 to 4 weeks to prevent withdrawal symptoms [67]. Although midazolam concentrations decline relatively slowly after an infusion is discontinued, slow reduction of the infusion rate is preferred to abrupt discontinuation. This approach permits careful reappraisal of the patient's underlying condition to avoid a sudden return of agitation, requiring reloading of the sedative agent and a general setback to the patients' progress [66]. The weaning process begins by slowly decreasing the intravenous infusion rate, transitioning to subcutaneous or oral administration [67].

In pediatric patients, tapering can be accomplished with the use of continuous subcutaneous administration, while eliminating the need for intravenous access [6,66]. The advantage is removal of central venous access and elimination of the need for repeated needle sticks to maintain peripheral intravenous access. Concentrated solutions of midazolam (2.5–5 mg/mL) are used so that the maximum infusion rates do not exceed 3 mL per hour. Local anesthetic creams can be placed over the anticipated subcutaneous cannulation. Areas suitable for subcutaneous administration include the subclavicular region, abdomen, deltoid, or anterior aspect of the thigh. Either a standard 22-gauge intravenous cannula or a 23-gauge butterfly needle is inserted into the subcutaneous tissue. The site should be changed every 7 days or sooner if erythema develops [67].

The change from intravenous midazolam to long-acting oral sedatives, such as lorazepam, should take into account the difference in potency of the two drugs (midazolam/lorazepam = 1:2), and the half-life (midazolam/lorazepam = 1:6). After the second oral dose of lorazepam, the intravenous midazolam infusion should be decreased by 50%. After the third oral dose, midazolam is decreased by another 50% and then discontinued after the fourth oral dose [67].

When analgesics and BZDs are administered concomitantly, withdrawal from opioids in addition to BZDs must be addressed. Initiation of long-acting opioids, such as methadone, may facilitate weaning from intravenous opioids [2]. When changing from intravenous fentanyl to oral methadone, for example, one should consider the difference in potency of the two drugs (fentanyl/methadone = 100:1); half-life (fentanyl/methadone = 1:75–100); and the oral bioavailability of methadone (75%–80%). Increasing the dose to compensate for the decreased oral bioavailability of methadone is not needed for prevention of withdrawal symptoms. Cross-tolerance of opioids is not 100%, so that changing from one opioid to another may result in a decrease in the total dose required when calculated on a standard potency ratio. The initial oral methadone dose should equal the total daily intravenous fentanyl dose. After the second oral dose of methadone, the fentanyl infusion should be decreased by 50%, another 50% after the third dose, and discontinued after the fourth dose. Opioid withdrawal symptoms are treated with rescue doses of immediate-release morphine. The 24-hour total morphine dose is then added to the next day's methadone dose. Methadone doses are adjusted this way every 72 hours until the patient is stable and showing no signs of withdrawal. If excessive sedation occurs, the methadone dose should be reduced by 10% to 20% until the sedation subsides. The oral methadone dose should be tapered by 20% on a weekly basis. At this rate, the opioid should be discontinued within 5 to 6 weeks. BZDs for opioid withdrawal should be limited to the treatment of seizures and extreme irritability and not as a replacement for opioid therapy.

Clonidine, an α_2-adrenergic agonist, may have a role in the treatment of opioid withdrawal. α_2-Adrenergic receptors mediate part of their pharmacologic actions through the activation of the same potassium channel as opioid receptors. In pediatric patients, subcutaneous administration of concentrated solutions of fentanyl (25–50 µg/mL) may also be used to help wean patients from opioid infusions [67].

There are limited published data for prevention of propofol dependence and withdrawal syndrome. With long-term use, abrupt discontinuation of the infusion should be avoided [25]. If propofol withdrawal syndrome is suspected, the previous infusion rate should be restarted before withdrawal symptoms occur. The infusion rate may then be decreased by approximately 10% every 6 hours if tolerated by the patient [27]. If withdrawal symptoms reappear, increasing the dosage or duration of the infusion may be warranted. Unfortunately, consensus is still lacking on the ap-

propriate propofol tapering strategy in long-term ICU sedation and further work is needed in this area.

Because of the pharmacologic nature and Food and Drug Administration indication, short-term use of less than 24 hours of DEX may require no tapering strategy for drug discontinuation. Data are still lacking; abrupt discontinuation of chronic DEX infusion may trigger withdrawal symptoms similar to those reported for clonidine. Currently, guidelines on how to taper off DEX have not been established and further work is required to determine the appropriate tapering strategy for DEX after chronic administration [1].

Summary

Tolerance and withdrawal associated with sedative use concern health care providers in the ICU setting. To understand fully the mechanisms of tolerance and withdrawal, it is essential to be knowledgeable of the pharmacology for each sedative. In addition to the manifestations of tolerance and withdrawal, altered pharmacokinetic and pharmacodynamic properties of sedatives and analgesics in critically ill patients can induce complications. Tolerance can occur with all sedatives but more rapidly with BZD than with propofol and DEX. Certain factors (outpatient medication, social history, alcohol abuse, chronic exposure, increased drug clearance, and target receptor desensitization) may contribute to the development of tolerance. The onset of withdrawal syndrome from sedatives ranges from hours to days during the weaning period and this phenomenon tends to occur more frequently with higher doses of sedative use and chronic administration. In general, treatment of withdrawal syndrome is prevention and avoidance of abrupt discontinuation of therapy. Collaboration among the health care team for proper weaning from sedatives and analgesics reduces the risk of withdrawal symptoms. In short-term use, weaning can be done rapidly, whereas in prolonged administration weaning may take longer, up to 4 weeks. Other strategies to enhance the weaning process, especially in pediatrics, can include using subcutaneous or oral administration and changing to a longer-acting sedative while slowly tapering off a short-acting agent. A similar approach may also apply to discontinuation of an opioid but equal potency of opioids should be guaranteed when substituting one agent for another. α_2-Receptor agonists (clonidine and DEX) are also useful in facilitating opioid and sedative withdrawal. Further research is needed to understand better the development of tolerance and to determine the most clinically and cost-effective approach in weaning therapy for commonly used sedatives.

References

[1] Jacobi J, Fraser GL, Coursin DB, et al. Clinical practice guidelines for the sustained use of sedatives and analgesics in the critically ill adult. Crit Care Med 2002;30:119–41.

[2] Taylor D. Iatrogenic drug dependence: a problem in intensive care? Intensive Crit Care Nurs 1999;15: 95–100.

[3] World Health Organization. Lexicon of alcohol and drug terms published by the World Health Organization. Available at: http://www.who.int/substance_abuse/terminology/who_lexicon/en/. Accessed December 27, 2004.

[4] Puntillo K, Casella V, Reid M. Opioid and benzodiazepine tolerance and dependence: application of theory to critical care practice. Heart Lung 1997;26:317–24.

[5] Robb ND, Hargrave SA. Tolerance to intravenous midazolam as a result of oral benzodiazepine therapy: a potential problem for the provision of conscious sedation in dentistry. Anesth Pain Control Dent 1993; 2:94–7.

[6] Tobias JD. Subcutaneous administration of fentanyl and midazolam to prevent withdrawal after prolonged sedation in children. Crit Care Med 1999;27:2262–5.

[7] Fonsmark L, Rasmussen YH, Carl P. Occurrence of withdrawal in critically ill sedated children. Crit Care Med 1999;27:196–9.

[8] Marx CM, Rosenberg DI, Ambuel B, et al. Pediatric intensive care sedation: survey of fellowship training programs. Pediatrics 1993;91:369–78.

[9] Wagner BKJ, O'Hara DA. Pharmacokinetics and pharmacodynamics of sedatives and analgesics in the treatment of agitated critically ill patients. Clin Pharmacokinet 1997;33:426–53.

[10] Jacqz-Aigrain E, Burtin P. Clinical pharmacokinetics of sedatives in neonates. Clin Pharmacokinet 1996;31: 423–43.

[11] Coldwell SE, Kaufman E, Milgrom P, et al. Acute tolerance and reversal of the motor control effects of midazolam. Pharmacol Biochem Behav 1998;59: 537–45.

[12] Kroboth PD, Smith RB, Erb RJ. Tolerance to alprazolam after intravenous bolus and continuous infusion: psychomotor and EEG effects. Clin Pharmacol Ther 1988;43:270–7.

[13] Sury MRJ, Billingham I, Russell GN, et al. Acute benzodiazepine withdrawal syndrome after midazolam infusions in children. Crit Care Med 1989;17: 301–2.

[14] Kunkel EJ, Rodgers C, DeMaria PA, et al. Use of high dose benzodiazepines in alcohol and sedative withdrawal delirium. Gen Hosp Psychiatry 1997;19: 286–93.

[15] Wijdicks E, Sharborough F. New-onset seizures in critically ill patients. Neurology 1993;43:1042–3.

[16] Carnevale FA, Ducharme C. Adverse reactions to the withdrawal of opioids and benzodiazepines in paediatric intensive care. Intensive Crit Care Nurs 1997;13: 181–8.

[17] Bergman I, Steeves M, Burckart G, et al. Reversible neurologic abnormalities associated with prolonged intravenous midazolam and fentanyl administration. J Pediatr 1991;119:644–9.

[18] van Engelen BGM, Gimbrere JS, Booy LH. Benzodiazepine withdrawal reaction in two children following discontinuation of sedation with midazolam. Ann Pharmacother 1993;27:579–81.

[19] Rosen DA, Rosen KR. Midazolam for sedation in the paediatric intensive care unit. Intensive Care Med 1991;17:S15–9.

[20] Hantson P, Clemesssy J, Baud F. Withdrawal syndrome following midazolam infusion. Intensive Care Med 1995;21:190–1.

[21] Finley PR, Nolan Jr PE. Precipitation of benzodiazepine withdrawal following sudden discontinuation of midazolam. DICP 1989;23:151–2.

[22] Franck LS, Naughton I, Winter I. Opioid and benzodiazepine withdrawal symptoms in paediatric intensive care patients. Intensive Crit Care Nurs 2004;20: 344–51.

[23] Brown C, Albrecht R, Pettit H, et al. Opioid and benzodiazepine withdrawal syndrome in adult burn patients. Am Surg 2000;66:367–71.

[24] Cammarano WB, Pittet JF, Weitz S, et al. Acute withdrawal syndrome related to the administration of analgesic and sedative medications in adult intensive care unit patients. Crit Care Med 1998;26:674–84.

[25] Mirenda J, Broyles G. Propofol as used for sedation in the ICU. Chest 1995;108:539–48.

[26] Fulton B, Sorkin EM. Propofol: an overview of its pharmacology and a review of its clinical efficacy in intensive care sedation. Drugs 1995;50:636–57.

[27] Cawley MJ, Guse TM, Laroia A, et al. Propofol withdrawal syndrome in an adult patient in thermal injury. Pharmacotherapy 2003;23:933–9.

[28] Buckley PM. Propofol in patients needing long-term sedation in intensive care: an assessment of the development of tolerance. A pilot study. Intensive Care Med 1997;23:969–74.

[29] Boyle WA, Shear JM, White PF, et al. Tolerance and hyperlipemia during long-term sedation with propofol. Anesthesiology 1990;73:A245.

[30] Foster SJ, Buckley PM. A retrospective review of two years' experience with propofol in one intensive care unit. J Drug Dev 1989;2(Suppl 2):73–4.

[31] Diprivan prescribing information. Wilmington (DE): AstraZeneca; 2004. Available at: http://www.astrazeneca-us.com/pi/diprivan.pdf. Accessed December 28, 2004.

[32] Setlock M, Palmisano B. Tolerance does not develop to propofol used repeatedly for radiation therapy in children. Anesth Analg 1992;74:S278.

[33] Setlock MA, Palmisano BW, Berens RJ, et al. Tolerance to propofol generally does not develop in pediatric patients undergoing radiation therapy. Anesthesiology 1996;85:207–9.

[34] Deer TR, Rich GF. Propofol tolerance in a pediatric patient. Anesthesiology 1992;77:828–9.

[35] Keidan I, Perel A, Shabtai EL, et al. Children undergoing repeated exposures for radiation therapy do not develop tolerance to propofol: clinical and bispectral index data. Anesthesiology 2004;100:251–4.

[36] Mayhew JF, Abouleish AE. Lack of tolerance to propofol. Anesthesiology 1996;85:1209.

[37] Valente JF, Anderson GL, Branson RD, et al. Disadvantages of prolonged propofol sedation in the critical care unit. Crit Care Med 1994;22:710–2.

[38] Au J, Walker WS, Scott DHT. Withdrawal syndrome after propofol infusion. Anesthesia 1990;45:741–2.

[39] Victory RA, Magee D. A case of convulsion after propofol anaesthesia. Anaesthesia 1988;43:904.

[40] Imray JM, Hay A. Withdrawal syndrome after propofol. Anaesthesia 1991;46:704.

[41] Walder B, Tramer MR, Seeck M. Seizure-like phenomena and propofol. Neurology 2002;58:1327–32.

[42] Marik PE, Varon J. The management of status epilepticus. Chest 2004;126:582–91.

[43] Bhana N, Goa KL, McClellan KJ. Dexmedetomidine. Drugs 2000;59:263–8.

[44] Virtanen R, Savola JM, Saano V, et al. Characterization of the selectivity, specificity and potency of medetomidine as an alpha 2-adrenoceptor agonist. Eur J Pharmacol 1988;150:9–14.

[45] Precedex prescribing information. North Chicago (IL): Abbott Laboratories; 2004. Available at: http://www.astrazeneca-us.com/pi/diprivan.pdf. Accessed December 28, 2004.

[46] Khan ZP, Ferguson CN, Jones RM. Alpha-2 and imidazoline receptor agonists. Anaesthesia 1999;54:146–65.

[47] Maze M, Scarfini C, Cavaliere F. New agents for sedation in the intensive care unit. Crit Care Clin 2001; 17:881–97.

[48] Paalzow G. Development of tolerance to the analgesic effect of clonidine in rats: cross-tolerance to morphine. Naunyn Schmiedebergs Arch Pharmacol 1978; 304:1–4.

[49] Yaksh TL, Reddy SV. Studies in the primate on the analgetic effects associated with intrathecal actions of opiates, alpha-adrenergic agonists and baclofen. Anesthesiology 1981;54:451–67.

[50] Reid K, Hayashi Y, Guo TZ, et al. Chronic administration of an alpha 2 adrenergic agonist desensitizes rats to the anesthetic effects of dexmedetomidine. Pharmacol Biochem Behav 1994;47:171–5.

[51] Reid K, Hayashi Y, Hsu J, et al. Chronic treatment with dexmedetomidine desensitizes α_2-adrenergic signal transduction. Pharmacol Biochem Behav 1997;57: 63–71.

[52] Hayashi Y, Guo TZ, Maze M. Desensitization to the behavioral effects of alpha 2-adrenergic agonists in rats. Anesthesiology 1995;82:954–62.

[53] Jones CR, Giembcyz M, Hamilton CA, et al. Desensitization of platelet alpha 2-adrenoceptors after short term infusions of adrenoceptor agonist in man. Clin Sci (Lond) 1986;70:147–53.

[54] Rabin BC, Reid K, Guo TZ, et al. Sympatholytic and minimum anesthetic concentration-sparing responses are preserved in rats rendered tolerant to the hypnotic and analgesic action of dexmedetomidine, a selective alpha(2)-adrenergic agonist. Anesthesiology 1996;85: 565–73.

[55] Bol CJJG, Danhof M, Stanski DR, et al. Pharmacokinetic-pharmacodynamic characterization of the cardiovascular, hypnotic, EEG and ventilatory responses to dexmedetomidine in the rat. J Pharmacol Exp Ther 1997;283:1051–8.

[56] Hayashi Y, Guo TZ, Maze M. Hypnotic and analgesic effects of the α_2-adrenergic agonist dexmedetomidine in morphine-tolerant rats. Anesth Analg 1996;83: 606–10.

[57] Kalso EA, Sullivan AF, McQuay HJ, et al. Cross-tolerance between *Mu* opioid and alpha-2 adrenergic receptors, but not between *Mu* and *Delta* opioid receptors in the spinal cord of the rat. J Pharmacol Exp Ther 1993;256:551–8.

[58] Finkel JC, Elrefai A. The use of dexmedetomidine to facilitate opioid and benzodiazepine detoxification in an infant. Anesth Analg 2004;98:1658–9.

[59] Maccioli GA. Dexmedetomidine to facilitate drug withdrawal. Anesthesiology 2003;98:575–7.

[60] Multz AS. Prolonged dexmedetomidine infusion as an adjunct in treating sedation-induced withdrawal. Anesth Analg 2003;96:1054–5.

[61] Angst MS, Koppert W, Pahl I, et al. Short-term infusion of the mu-opioid agonist remifentanil in humans causes hyperalgesia during withdrawal. Pain 2003;106: 49–57.

[62] Compton P, Charuvastra VC, Ling W. Pain intolerance in opioid-maintained former opiate addicts: effect of long-acting maintenance agent. Drug Alcohol Depend 2001;63:139–46.

[63] Tilson HA, Rech RH, Stolman S. Hyperalgesia during withdrawal as a means of measuring the degree of dependence in morphine dependent rats. Psychopharmacologia 1973;28:287–300.

[64] VonVoigtlander PF, Lewis RA. A withdrawal hyperalgesia test for physical dependence: evaluation of mu and mixed-partial opioid agonists. J Pharmacol Methods 1983;10:277–82.

[65] Davies MF, Haimor F, Lighthall G, et al. Dexmedetomidine fails to cause hyperalgesia after cessation of chronic administration. Anesth Analg 2003;96: 195–200.

[66] Shafer A. Complications of sedation with midazolam in the intensive care unit and a comparison with other sedative regimens. Crit Care Med 1998;26:947–56.

[67] Tobias JD. Tolerance, withdrawal, and physical dependency after long-term sedation and analgesia of children in the pediatric intensive care unit. Crit Care Med 2000;28:2122–32.

ELSEVIER
SAUNDERS

Crit Care Nurs Clin N Am 17 (2005) 225–237

CRITICAL CARE
NURSING CLINICS
OF NORTH AMERICA

Sleep Deprivation and Psychosocial Impact in Acutely Ill Cancer Patients

Roberta Kaplow, RN, PhD, CCNS, CCRN

Nell Hodgson Woodruff School of Nursing, Emory University, 1520 Clifton Road NE, Atlanta, GA 30322-4207, USA

There is universal agreement that sleep is an important factor related to health and quality of life [1,2]. Sleep disturbances are common and are a source of distress among patients with cancer [1–15]. This article summarizes the problem of sleep in patients with cancer, and reviews the types, prevalence, etiology, risk factors, clinical sequelae, and management of sleep disturbances. Nursing implications and research in the area are described.

Despite the universal agreement that there is a high prevalence of sleep disturbances in patients with cancer and that sleep is essential, there is a paucity of data available regarding this problem. Further compounding the problem is the fact that health care providers do not inquire about or provide interventions for patients' sleep problems [1,8,16].

The process of sleep

To appreciate sleep disturbances in patients with cancer, it is essential to have an understanding of the process of sleep. There are two processes of sleep: process S and process C. Process S is involved with sleep homeostasis and the drive to sleep. The drive to sleep depends on prior waking or sleeping. The relationship is intuitive. The longer one is awake, the greater the drive to sleep. For example, if a person awakens at 5 AM, it is likely that person will get sleepy around 10 PM because of being awake for many hours. What dissipates this drive is sleep.

Similarly, the longer one sleeps, there is a decrease in the drive to sleep, resulting in awakening [17]. Process C influences sleep propensity and waking, involves circadian rhythms, and is a sinusoidal rhythm. The rhythms are driven by a clock mechanism in the brain [17].

Processes S and C work in tandem. When one is asleep, process C is low; when one is awake, process C increases. Process S increases during the day, building up the need for sleep. Concomitantly, process C counterbalances the need to sleep, thereby keeping one awake. In the early evening, process C decreases as body temperature decreases. As temperature drops and process S increases, one goes to sleep [17].

Research has shown that normal sleep has two states: rapid eye movement (REM) and non-REM. In non-REM sleep, electroencephalogram activity becomes increasingly synchronous, mental activity is increasingly fragmented, and muscle tone is reduced. A common definition of non-REM sleep is a relatively inactive brain in a movable body [17,18]. REM sleep is characterized by electroencephalogram activation, muscle atony, bursts of eye movement, dreaming, and autonomic variability (increases in heart rate, respiration and blood pressure, cerebral blood flow, decreased temperature regulation). The common definition of REM sleep is a highly activated brain in a paralyzed body [17,18]. This entire process is relevant because sleep regulatory processes are disturbed with cancer. Processes S and C are disrupted in cancer patients for a variety of reasons. The reader is encouraged to explore the sleep literature for a more in-depth understanding of sleep processes.

E-mail address: rkaplow@emory.edu

Types of sleep disorders in patients with cancer

There are varying data regarding the types of sleep disturbances and sequelae experienced by patients with cancer. In an extensive review of the literature, Clark and coworkers [3] categorized these disorders. Groupings included general (including sleep problems, sleep disturbances, and sleep difficulty); sleep disorders (including insomnia [difficulty in initiating or maintaining sleep] [1], somnolence syndrome, and nightmares); and specific sleep-wake descriptors (sleep quality, decreased sleep efficiency [the ratio of total sleep time/time in bed] [1], increased sleep latency, decreased sleep latency, difficulty going to sleep, wake after sleep onset, frequent awakenings, increased nightmare awakenings, wake for a long time, difficulty getting back to sleep, waking too early, reduced sleep, increased hours of sleep, increased nighttime sleep, increased daytime napping, overly sleepy, and increased daytime sleepiness).

Other researchers have reported the prevalence of several types of sleep problems. Of those reported, insomnia is the sleep disturbance that has been reported most often [5,7,8,19,20]. Many of the other disorders corroborate the report by Clark and coworkers [3]. Some of these include excessive fatigue [5,19], restless leg syndrome [5], excessive sleepiness [5], increased amount of time spent in bed [19], increased amount of time napping [19], dreaming more than usual [5], frightening or unpleasant dreams [5,16], use of tranquilizers or sleeping pills [5,19], problems initiating sleep [6,20], problems maintaining sleep [6,20], difficulty sleeping in general [9], early morning awakenings [16,20], sleeping during unusual hours [7,16], sleeping fewer hours [16], trouble getting back to sleep [16], and multiple awakenings [5,19]. Some patients experienced problems with sleep latency and efficiency [4,19,21], whereas others reported difficulty with sleep onset and maintenance [7]. In one study, 18% of patients with cancer reported they were more likely to doze during the day than usual and 40% reported they were less likely to sleep at night [15]. In another study, a convenience sample of patients with cancer reported poorer sleep quality specifically manifested by difficulty falling asleep, shorter and less efficient nocturnal sleep, and increased use of sleep medications as compared with healthy subjects [20].

Prevalence of sleep disorders in patients with cancer

Numerous studies have been conducted that have focused on sleep disturbances in cancer patients. Data

reveal disparate results, with incidence ranging from 18% to 95% [3,7,8,15,16,21–27]. Reports range from anecdotal experience [23] to clinical studies. The literature is variable in terms of how prevalence of sleep disorders is described.

There are contrasting data regarding sleep disturbances in patients with cancer. For example, Kaye and coworkers [22] reported that cancer patients had more sleep maintenance problems than a comparison of cardiac patients and a control group. Conversely, Lamb [28] found no difference in sleeping patterns between hospitalized patients with cancer and those patients with nonmalignant diseases.

Differences in prevalence are reported related to site-specific cancers. Patients with breast cancer have a high prevalence of insomnia [5,8], reported as high as 53% [4]. Similarly, patients with lung cancer have a high prevalence of sleep problems [5,12], reported as high as 79% in one study sample [4]. In another study, patients with breast or lung cancer slept longer than patients with a history of insomnia. The patients with lung cancer in this sample had lower more disturbed sleep and compensated by increasing their time spent in bed [4]. In a third study of lung cancer patients, 36% of the study sample claimed that they were poor sleepers [12].

Researchers have also reported prevalence of sleep disturbances in relation to cancer treatment modalities. Beszterczey and Lipowski [29] revealed that of 47 patients who received radiation therapy, 45% averaged <50 hours of sleep per week and 23% averaged <40 hours of sleep per week. Other data suggest that the sleep disturbances reported were not related to diagnosis, stage of disease, or treatment modality [16].

Mills and Graci [30] suggest that sleep disturbances that are experienced by patients with cancer may occur at different phases of the disease trajectory (eg, time of diagnosis, during treatment, during the end-of-life phase). Not only are sleep disturbances problematic on diagnosis and treatment, but also data suggest that symptoms persist many months following treatment. In one study, 75% of patients had problems lasting for at least 6 months [5] and as long as 2 to 5 years following treatment [31–33]. In another study, patients reported sleep disturbances 6 months before diagnosis and up to 18 months postdiagnosis [5].

The importance of sleep

Patients often find sleep as a reprieve from the distress, pain, and fatigue associated with illness [34].

It has been demonstrated that inadequate sleep can impact clinical outcomes. Sleep disturbances have been identified as a source of distress and having a significant impact on a cancer patient's quality of life [5,7,10,13,35–37].

From a cancer defense perspective, there are data that connect sleep and activity of natural killer cells, which could have a role in the immune system's defense against cancer cells [5,34,38]. Further, it is suggested that sleep disturbances can impact a patient's tolerance to cancer treatment.

Alleviating sleep disturbances may also eliminate the harmful effects on a patient's emotional, cognitive, and physical functioning [5]. Data suggest that reduced sleep has a negative effect on daytime mood and performance [7,33,36,39,40]. In addition, unrelenting sleep disturbances increase the risk of the patient in the general population developing anxiety or depression [7,36,41,42]. In patients with cancer, data suggest a relationship between sleep disturbances and fatigue, pain, wound healing, and mental health [43], and have contributed to decreased functional status [44]. Patients with metastatic breast cancer have identified sleep as an important health outcome [45].

Etiologic factors

Sleep disturbances experienced by patients with cancer have been attributed to a number of factors [35]. Several factors exist alone or in combination. It is customary for health care providers and patients with cancer alike to blame psychologic factors as the cause of sleep disturbances [4]. Other factors, however, have also been implicated. Savard and Morin [8] divided the etiologic factors of sleep disturbance into three categories: (1) predisposing factors, (2) precipitating factors, and (3) perpetuating factors.

Predisposing factors

Predisposing factors increase a patient's susceptibility to develop sleep disturbances [8]. Factors include female gender, aging, and personal and family history of insomnia [46]. Patients with sleep disturbances before diagnosis often have these disturbances persist or worsen on diagnosis [1]. Presence of coexisting psychiatric disorders can lead to the development of sleep disturbances [47].

There are inconsistent data regarding the relationship between sleep disturbances and gender in patients with cancer [3]. Results of one study revealed a significant correlation between the presence of sleep disturbances and gender [48]. Results of another study, however, revealed no significant correlation [9]. Studies exploring the relationship between age and sleep disturbances in patients with cancer have revealed disparate results. Some data suggest older patients receiving antineoplastic therapies experienced fewer sleep disturbances than younger patients [5,9,48]. Conversely, some earlier data suggest no relationship between age and sleep disturbances in patients with cancer [49]. Some data suggest that the risk of insomnia, one of the most frequently reported sleep disturbances in patients with cancer, also increases in people who are unemployed and people who live alone [1,34,50,51].

Precipitating factors

Precipitating factors are conditions that can trigger the development of sleep disturbances [8]. Some precipitating factors include pain, the tumor itself, treatment modalities, the patient's environment, lifestyle, altered hormones, cytokines, altered activity and rest, and psychiatric issues related to cancer diagnosis or treatment.

Pain

It has been suggested that pain plays an important role in the development of sleep disturbances in patients with cancer [5,6,19,21,32,52]. In one study, 37% of patients with cancer who had pain reported problems with sleep latency and 65% reported trouble staying asleep through the night [53]. Likewise, 56% of another group of patients with cancer reported that pain hindered sleep [54]. In two additional studies, 58% and 61% of patients reported they wake up because of pain [55,56]. As expected, data further support an inverse relationship between pain intensity and amount of sleep [57].

It has been further demonstrated that sleep disturbances lower a patient's pain threshold. This effect is reversed with the resolution of sleep disturbances [58]. Studies have demonstrated an improvement in sleep when pain is controlled [59–61]. Pain causes problems with initiation of sleep and sleep maintenance [8]. Other data, however, revealed no significant relationship between pain and presence of sleep disturbances [4].

Studies have yielded disparate results regarding the relationship between pain and sleep disturbances [3]. Beszterczey and Lipowski [29] evaluated the presence of sleep disturbance and pain in patients who were receiving radiotherapy. They reported no correlation between pain and sleep disturbances.

Similarly, Engstrom and coworkers [16], who evaluated patients with breast and lung cancer, found no correlation between these two variables. Conversely, several researchers reported increased pain with increased disruption in sleep [53,62–65]. One study evaluating patients with breast cancer and one evaluating patients with lung cancer reported a significant relationship between pain and sleep disturbance [1,5]. Consistent with these latter findings, it has also been concluded that pain control decreases the prevalence and severity of sleep disturbances [66]. Finally, patients with sleep disturbances have reported heightened pain perception [56].

Tumor effects

Tumors and associated responses may be sources of sleep disturbances. For example, patients with brainstem tumors, head and neck cancer, or pancreatic carcinoma have reported sleep disturbances [7]. Dyspnea in patients with a primary pulmonary lesion or pulmonary metastasis can lead to sleep disturbances [4,6,7,19]. This is believed to be related to feelings of breathlessness and increased arousal from the anxiety associated with feeling breathless [32]. Gastrointestinal disturbances associated with cancer, such as nausea, vomiting, diarrhea, or constipation, disrupt sleep [32,52].

Treatment-related causes

The treatment of cancer places patients at risk for sleep disturbance. For example, emotional and physiologic effects, and functional loss following surgical intervention can cause emotional distress. In one study, recent cancer surgery was identified as a variable associated with an increased risk of insomnia [5]. Chemotherapy, radiotherapy, hormones, biotherapy, psychotropic drugs, and corticosteroids can precipitate sleep disturbances [1,7,19,32,35]. Many other medications hinder normal sleep [32]. These include bronchodilators, methyldopa, propranolol, central nervous system stimulants, monoamine oxidase inhibitors, fluoxetine, protriptyline, and bupropion. Antidepressants with sedating properties can cause daytime sleepiness; decreased REM sleep; and an increase in total sleep time [34] (the amount of actual sleep in a sleep episode) [1]. Antiemetics, such as $5-HT_3$ receptor antagonists, which are the mainstay of prevention and treatment of chemotherapy-induced nausea and vomiting, can cause a decrease in REM sleep. Opioids can cause a decrease in total sleep time and REM sleep, and increase drowsiness [32,34]. Anxiolytics, such as benzodiazepines, can cause a decrease in REM sleep [34].

Chemotherapy is associated with the development of sleep disturbances. This has been attributed to anxiety related to treatment, side effects of treatment, and use of antiemetics [1,8] demonstrated in patients who have undergone bone marrow transplantation [67]. Patients in one study who received chemotherapy as treatment for breast cancer reported exacerbated or newly developed sleep disturbances, possibly a result of antiemetics given for chemotherapy-induced nausea or the development of menopausal symptoms. In this same study, the patients who had undergone a lumpectomy developed an increased risk for sleep disturbances [1]. The relationship between the development of sleep disturbance and administration of chemotherapy has also been supported in other studies [68–70].

Radiation therapy is also associated with the development of sleep disturbances [8]. In one study, women who received radiation therapy for breast cancer had a higher incidence of sleep disturbances in comparison with those who did not have radiation therapy [47]. These findings were corroborated in patients being treated with radiation therapy for bone metastasis [52].

Reports of the presence of sleep disturbances are similar in patients receiving radiation therapy as with chemotherapy [29,52]. It has been suggested that the etiology of sleep disturbances in this patient population may be cytokine levels [34,71]. Data suggest that there is an increased level of interleukin-1 in patients during the first 4 weeks of therapy [72].

Hormonal therapy has also been implicated in the development of sleep disturbances in patients with cancer. This is believed to be caused by side effects of therapy (ie, menopausal symptoms in women and androgen-deprivation therapy in men with prostate cancer) [32]. Disparate results exist related to hormonal therapy as an etiologic factor of sleep disturbances [1].

In a study of patients with breast cancer, the presence and severity of hot flashes and night sweats increased sleep disturbances [31]. These findings were later corroborated by other researchers [70,73–77]. It has been suggested that the stage of disease, time elapsed since diagnosis, the recurrence of disease, associated side effects of cancer treatment modalities, and cancer-associated comorbidities may result in sleep disturbances [1]. It has been further suggested in one study of patients with breast and lung cancer who had recent treatment and experienced an increase in fatigue and hypersomnolence [5].

Although often prescribed for management of sleep disturbances, anxiolytics and antidepressants can have a negative effect on aspects of sleep [3].

These same authors list four other categories of drugs that are frequently administered to patients with cancer that can cause sleep disturbances: (1) analgesics (including opioids and nonsteroidal anti-inflammatory agents); (2) antiemetics (ie, dopamine antagonists, anticholinergic agents, and 5-HT$_3$ antagonists); (3) corticosteroids; and (4) hypnotics. Two of the effects of analgesics are a decrease in REM sleep and decreased arousal [3]. Antidepressant administration causes a decrease in REM sleep and an increase in total sleep time. Dopamine antagonists cause drowsiness, sedation, and a decrease in REM sleep. Anticholinergic agents cause a delay in the onset of REM sleep and a decrease in REM sleep. The main effect of 5-HT$_3$ antagonists is drowsiness. One of the primary effects of anxiolytics is a decrease in REM sleep. Corticosteroids cause insomnia and bad dreams. Finally, hypnotics, such as benzodiazepines, cause a decrease in REM sleep [3].

Environmental factors

Sleep disturbances reportedly are encountered in the home and the hospital setting [6]. It has been suggested that the presence of certain environmental stimuli can impact the onset of sleep. These include the presence of noise and light and room temperature [34,78]. Results, however, are inconclusive because three earlier studies have conflicting results. In two studies, patients with cancer who were at home reported sleep disturbances [22,29]. Similar results were reported in hospitalized patients [79]. Conversely, Lamb [28] reported no differences in sleep disturbances between patients with cancer who were at home versus those who were hospitalized.

Hospital admission is associated with the development of sleep disturbances [19,34,80]. This can be attributed to disruptions by staff rendering aspects of care, extreme environmental noise or lighting, or noise created by other patients. Sequelae of sleep disturbances associated with environmental factors are a decrease in total sleep and daytime napping [32].

Sheely [6] described the relationship between nocturnal disturbances and sleep length and quality of patients with cancer who were hospitalized. It was concluded that the greater number of nocturnal disturbances and the higher level of patient participation in care had a negative correlation with the quality of sleep.

Lifestyle factors

Alcohol intake is associated with frequent awakenings [19,34]. Caffeine and nicotine also have the potential to cause sleep disturbances [19,32,34].

Altered hormone secretion

Patients with cancer have variable levels of cortisol [34,81]. Fluctuating cortisol levels may alter circadian processes [34,82] and contribute to sleep disturbances experienced by cancer patients.

Cytokine production

Cytokines are small biologically active molecules that mediate and regulate inflammation [83]. Cytokines have been implicated in relation to sleep regulation [1]. Because cancer cells produce cytokines, it has been suggested that the daytime sleepiness reported by cancer patients may be attributed to increased levels of cytokines, specifically interleukin-1; tumor necrosis factor-α, which enhances non-REM sleep; and interferon, which reduces the amount of slow wave (non-REM) and REM sleep [27,34].

Altered activity and rest

It has been suggested that patients with cancer experiencing a change in their sequence of activities of daily living (eg, timing of meals, including activity in their day-to-day life, and social interaction) may be prone to sleep disturbances [34,84]. Further, taking naps during the day, often reported in patients with cancer during treatment, has been reported to cause sleep disturbances at night [34].

Psychologic factors

A cancer diagnosis is often associated with a number of stressors that can lead to sleep disturbances. Psychologic factors that can cause sleep disturbances may include onset of a stressful life event, such as cancer; concerns regarding cancer treatment and impact on the family; depression; and anxiety. Depression and anxiety are two of the more common psychologic responses to a cancer diagnosis. These responses can result in sleep disturbances [1,5–7, 13,19,32,52]. Patients with depression characteristically awaken during the night and early morning. Patients with anxiety traditionally have sleep latency [7]. This relationship is inconsistently reported in the literature. Results of two studies indicated a positive correlation between presence of depression and sleep disturbances in patients with cancer [9,85]. Other factors, such as debility and concern about the future, have been cited as having a causal relationship with sleep disturbances [15].

Delirium, another psychiatric condition that might develop as a result of cancer, is also associated with development of sleep disturbances [7,8]. Delirium may be caused by brain metastasis, fever, metabolic derangements, or medications [7].

Perpetuating factors

Perpetuating factors contribute to the sustainability of the sleep disturbances over time [8]. Although some believe that sleep disturbances are short-lived and normal consequences to the diagnosis and treatment of cancer and that the disturbances dissipate over time, it is possible for sleep disturbances to become a chronic problem. These patients compensate by spending more time in bed, napping, and have erratic sleep-wake cycles [8]. Patients with sleep disturbances are inclined to partake in activities that interfere with sleep (eg, reading, listening to music, or watching television in bed).

Clinical sequelae

Sleep disturbances can result in serious physical and emotional consequences and can cause a number of debilitating conditions that can affect functioning during daytime hours and quality of life [9,34]. Researchers have described the impact of physical and psychosocial functioning, mood, symptom distress, and survival from cancer as potential sequelae to long-term sleep disturbances [8,49,86–88]. Physiologic consequences of sleep disturbances that have been reported include headache, diarrhea, stomach discomfort, palpitations, and nonspecific pain [8]. Patients with sleep disturbances have verbalized concerns about getting inadequate rest and reported seeking more medical consultations and hospitalizations than patients who sleep well [8,89].

Another consequence of sleep disturbances can be excessive daytime sleepiness (the inability to maintain the alert-awake state) [1]. Insomnia (difficulty in initiating or maintaining sleep) [1] has been reported to have a negative impact on concentration [5]. In addition, sleep disturbances can result in an increase in fatigability, irritability, aggressiveness, anxiety, and a decrease in pain tolerance [6,8,16], with fatigability being one of the most common complaints of patients with insomnia [8].

There is some preliminary evidence suggesting that sleep disturbances can impact morbidity and mortality of patients with cancer [8]. In a study of newly diagnosed patients with different types of cancer, patients with such symptoms as insomnia survived an average of 5 years less than patients without these symptoms [23]. This relationship needs further investigation.

Management of sleep disturbances in patients with cancer

Given the significant potential sequelae of sleep disturbances in patients with cancer, prompt recognition and management are essential [8]. There is universal agreement that management of sleep disturbances should focus on the underlying etiology, which should be promptly identified and treated [7,8,19,32].

Pharmacologic interventions

There are several alternatives in terms of pharmacologic intervention if indicated for the patient [7]. Data are inadequate for specific recommendations for pharmacologic interventions. Data do suggest, however, that health care providers should do a cost-benefit analysis in terms of side effects profile and effectiveness when prescribing or administering any agent [3].

In a sample of approximately 1600 patients with cancer, hypnotics were prescribed most commonly for patients who are experiencing sleep disturbances [19,90]. Others have also suggested the use of hypnotics [7,8,32]. Data from one study dating back 25 years suggested that of 1579 patients, 51% received a prescription for a psychotropic agent. Of those patients, 44% received the prescription as a sleep aid [91]. More recent studies revealed use of hypnotics in cancer patients ranged from 43% to 77% [3,92] during different phases of the disease trajectory. Of note, however, is this class of medications might not be the most effective category of medications to treat the sleep disturbances associated with a cancer diagnosis. Data further suggest that pharmacologic interventions may be beneficial on a short-term basis but may produce effects that are more harmful than beneficial [19].

In addition to hypnotics, benzodiazepines are frequently prescribed for patients with cancer with sleep disturbances [7,32]. There have been reports, however, of patient complaints of daytime sleepiness, confusion, cognitive and psychomotor impairment, dizziness, lightheadedness, and dose-dependent anterograde amnesia with use of some of these agents [7,8,32,91,93]. These side effects have a higher prevalence in the elderly. This is of clinical significance because many patients with cancer fall into this age bracket [8]. Data from a meta-analysis further suggest that use of benzodiazepines only increases the duration of sleep but insignificantly reduces sleep latency [8].

Use of sedating antidepressants to treat sleep disturbances in patients with cancer may also be indicated. Sedative-hypnotics (eg, barbiturates) or antidepressants are described in the literature as an alternative to benzodiazepines [7]. There are several risks associated with sedative-hypnotics including the risk of tolerance, abuse, dependence, and overdose. These agents are usually not beneficial in treating insomnia for patients who have already tried benzodiazepines [7,8], making these agents an unsuitable choice following benzodiazepine use.

If the underlying etiology of sleep disturbance in the patient with cancer is caused by a psychiatric disorder, psychotherapy and antidepressants may be indicated [8]. Administration of antidepressants may be helpful in patients with depression and for patients with potential for abuse or dependence on other drugs. Tricyclic antidepressants are frequently prescribed and have a sedating effect [7]. If the etiology is an anxiety disorder, patients may be treated with psychotherapy, anxiolytics, and behavioral techniques. Analgesics are indicated if the patient's sleep disturbance is caused by pain [7].

Given the many choices available for pharmacologic intervention for sleep disturbances, it is essential for the health care provider to individualize the decision of which medication to prescribe based on the patient, etiology of the sleep disturbance, expected amount of time the patient requires medication, and potential side effects [32].

Nonpharmacologic interventions

Pharmacologic intervention may not be indicated in all instances of sleep disturbances [7]. Reasons include patient preference, confusion, daytime sedation, and potential drug-drug interaction [7]. Several nonpharmacologic interventions have been developed and used to treat sleep disturbances for more than two decades. The methods that have been found most valuable for patients with cancer are stimulus control, sleep restriction, and the combination of a number of techniques. Other methods include relaxation and cognitive therapy [8]. Reports of hypnosis, biofeedback, autogenic training, and systematic desensitization being used in patients with cancer with sleep disturbances also appear in the literature [10].

Patient environment

Basic measures should be implemented to enhance sleep and rest, especially for those experiencing sleep disturbances. For example, noise can be controlled with the use of ear plugs and minimizing extraneous environmental noise. The room temperature should also be set at a comfortable level. If the room is too cold or hot, the patient may experience difficulty sleeping [7,19].

Avoidance of stimulants

It has been suggested that intake of stimulants, such as caffeine-containing products, should be avoided after lunchtime to avoid difficulty falling asleep at night [7,19,21,32]. Further, alcohol intake may result in sleep that is fragmented [7].

Sleep schedules

Establishing and maintaining a regular sleep-wake schedule is important to manage sleep disturbances associated with cancer. Hu and Silberfarb [7] listed rules of sleep hygiene (conditions and practices that promote continuous and effective sleep) [1]. These rules include (1) sleeping only as long as needed to feel refreshed but not longer; (2) waking at the same time each day regardless of how the patient slept during the night; (3) establishing an exercise routine, promote an environment conducive to sleep by minimizing noise, and establishing a comfortable room temperature; (4) having a bedtime snack to avoid bedtime hunger; (5) being aware of how napping during the day affects the patient; (6) avoiding stimulants and limiting ingestion of alcohol; and (7) turning on the light and engaging in an activity if unable to fall asleep. This latter suggestion helps avert some of the frustration or tension of being unable to sleep.

Another sleep expert identified similar measures for sleep hygiene for palliative care patients. Recommendations included (1) maintaining a regular sleep schedule; (2) avoiding unnecessary time in bed; (3) avoiding napping, especially in the late afternoon and evening; (4) keeping as active a daytime schedule as possible; (5) controlling environmental factors that may cause sleep disruptions, such as noise, stimulants, and medications; (6) avoiding lying in bed frustrated when unable to sleep (engage in another activity until feeling drowsy); (7) identify and address issues and concerns of the day before attempting to sleep; and (8) maintain pain relief with long-acting analgesics [12] and avoid taking diuretics in the evening if possible [19].

Relaxation techniques

Data suggest that behavioral interventions that have been used for over 20 years may be helpful in the management of sleep disturbances experienced by patients with cancer. Some techniques include muscle relaxation [10,15,94], somatic focusing, imagery, and cognitive-behavioral therapy [95]. The relaxation techniques aimed at minimizing cognitive arousal have been found to be effective in treating insomnia in patients with cancer [5,10,46].

Thomas [19] suggested a number of nonpharmacologic techniques to manage sleep disturbances. These included relaxation tapes; warm baths; back rubs; a daily routine of activities; decreasing sedentary activities; avoiding strenuous activities around bedtime; assuming a comfortable position for sleep; and using bed for sleeping only, not resting.

The use of combination therapies to promote sleep in patients with cancer shows promise. The Individualized Sleep Promotion Plan was evaluated over two phases: during treatment with chemotherapy for breast cancer and longitudinally over 1 year after treatment. Therapies included sleep hygiene, relaxation, stimulus control, and sleep restriction activities. Results were mixed in terms of efficacy of the program. Subjects of this study had scores 3.7 to 3.8 (out of 5) in terms of feeling refreshed on waking and sleep efficacy at 82% to 92%. These subjects also reported being awakened 10 to 11 times per night because of nightmares; taking naps during the daytime hours for 10 to 15 minutes; a total rest time of 7 to 8 hours; and sleep latency (time from lights out to the onset of sleep) [1] of less than 30 minutes [96].

Use and efficacy of many of these techniques is well documented in studies of noncancer patients. Data from one recent study of cancer survivors revealed that a six-session sleep therapy program including stimulus control therapy, relaxation, training, and other strategies aimed at decreasing cognitive-emotional arousal decreased the number of awakenings, time awake after sleep onset, and increased sleep efficiency, and sleep quality [86]. Further data are needed in patients with cancer with sleep disturbances [8].

Exercise program

Data from a recent study suggests that participation in an exercise program may improve sleep patterns. In this study, subjects participated in a cardiac rehabilitation program of exercise and education 2 days per week for 12 weeks. On completion of the program, patients reported significant improve-ments in their sleep patterns and quality of life [97]. Other sleep experts support the use of exercise to promote optimal sleep [9,21,97].

Information

A recent comparison study of patients with prostate cancer who were receiving radiotherapy was conducted to determine the efficacy of an educational intervention. The patients in the intervention group reported fewer sleep disturbances than the control group [3,98]. It is important, in general, for nurses to provide information to patients regarding the incidence of sleep disturbances in cancer and treatment and to devise a plan of care to help with management [99].

Expressive writing

In a study of patients with metastatic renal cell carcinoma, effects of expressive writing were evaluated. Patients in the intervention group were requested to express their deepest thoughts and feelings about cancer, whereas patients in the control group were asked to write about a more neutral topic on a health behavior, such as diet, physical activity, substance abuse, or sleep. Patients who participated in the expressive writing group reported higher sleep quality, sleep duration, and daytime functioning.

Mindfulness-based stress reduction

Recently, Shapiro and coworkers [100] evaluated the effectiveness of mindfulness-based stress reduction to treat sleep disturbances in patients who had been successfully treated for breast cancer. The women who received mindfulness-based stress reduction were taught meditative processes including awareness of body sensations, thoughts, and emotions; progressive movement of attention through the body; and stretches and postures. The control group participants had free choice over their selection of stress management techniques and were not given any instructions on use of the technique. Both groups reported feeling refreshed after sleep.

Psychotherapy

Sleep experts suggest that a brief period of psychotherapy may be helpful for patients with cancer who are experiencing sleep disturbances. Sessions can be used to assist the patient to ventilate fears and hopes related to the disease. The experts further advise that the sessions not primarily focus on the sleep disturbances and that therapists should focus the patient to discuss anxieties, conflicts, and disappointments, especially during the terminal phase of the disease [32].

Implications for nursing practice

The prevalence of sleep disturbances in patients with cancer and the clinical sequelae have significant implications for oncology nursing practice. Treatment of sleep disturbances can enhance a patient's quality of life [9,21] and reduce morbidity. It has also been suggested that minimizing sleep disturbances may enhance the immune status of a patient, thereby decreasing the risk of disease recurrence [21]. Further, the psychologic effects of chemotherapy, specifically depression and anxiety, are associated with sleep disturbances [9].

Identification of patients

Management of sleep disturbances begins with assessment for the problem [3,8,19,34]. Surprisingly, one of the primary reasons that sleep disturbances go unrecognized in patients is that they are not asked [32,101]. Data suggest that patients do not engage in self-help behaviors. They often do not share their distress with others [15,16]. Further compounding the problem is that even when sleep disturbances are reported, the problem is often dismissed, so patients do not get the attention needed to eliminate sleep disturbances [32]. The most logical way to determine if patients are experiencing sleep disturbances is by inquiring. Assessment of how easy it is for them to fall asleep, whether they stay asleep or awaken during the night, and how rested they feel in the morning provides a good foundation for determining presence of sleep disturbances [7]. A few assessment instruments have been developed to assist the clinician in identifying sleep disturbances [102,103]. Engstrom and coworkers [16] suggested questions that may be asked to assess sleep disturbances. (1) Do you have difficulty falling asleep? (2) Do you have difficulty staying asleep? (3) How many hours of sleep do you average each night? (4) Do you feel tired all of the time? When? How often? (5) Does inability to sleep cause your family to be awake at night? (6) What causes you to be unable to fall asleep? Stay asleep? Other important data points include exacerbating and alleviating factors, understanding the patient's normal sleep habits, and effectiveness of previous treatments [8].

Clinicians need to be cognizant of the fact that sleep needs vary among individuals. What may seemingly be enough sleep for the clinician may be inadequate for the patient [32]. Given the sequelae of sleep disturbances in patients with cancer, it is essential for nurses to develop strategies to encourage patients to report these problems and follow-up to ensure they are being addressed [3].

Identification of underlying cause

Identification of potential underlying causes should be attempted when patients experience sleep disturbances. Causes may be multifactorial (eg, physical, psychologic) and have been described. An assessment of lifestyle causes of sleep disturbances should also be made. This includes alcohol and caffeine consumption, use of nicotine, and evaluating the medications that the patient is currently receiving [32].

Sleep hygiene

Sateia and Silberfarb [32] suggest a number of strategies for sleep hygiene. Although they are suggestions for palliative care patients, many are translatable in other patients with cancer. The suggestions include

1. Maintain as regular a sleep-wake schedule as possible, particularly with respect to the hour of morning awakening
2. Avoid unnecessary time in bed during the day
3. Nap only as necessary and avoid napping in the late afternoon and evening whenever possible
4. Keep as active a daytime schedule as possible, including social contacts and light exercise when possible
5. Minimize nighttime sleep interruptions caused by medication, noise, or other environmental conditions
6. Avoid lying in bed for prolonged periods at night in an alert and frustrated or tense state
7. Remove unpleasant conditioned stimuli, such as clocks
8. Identify problems and concerns of the day before trying to sleep and address these issues with an active problem-solving approach

9. Avoid stimulating medication and other substances, particularly in the hours before bedtime
10. Maintain adequate pain relief through the night with long-acting analgesics
11. Use sleep medication as indicated and avoid overuse

Psychosocial support

Patients experience a number of symptoms during the cancer disease and treatment trajectory [16]. If sleep is disturbed, patients might attribute this to an expected part of cancer. Patients should be encouraged to report all symptoms experienced so symptoms can be ameliorated or palliated. Reporting of symptoms should be conducted in a therapeutic, accepting environment. Support should also be available for the family, who may be experiencing sleep disturbances along with the patient. Patients and families should be encouraged to report sleep disturbances and verbalize their concerns about them [16].

Scheduling of activities

Clustering of activities to minimize the number of times that a patient gets disturbed by health care workers helps to minimize sleep disturbances. This can be done by coordinating activities among disciplines and rescheduling nonessential activities [5]. It has been suggested that placing the patient in a room with a window that allows viewing without actually entering the room might minimize sleep disturbances [6].

Summary

Sleep disturbances are common in patients with cancer and have a negative impact on functioning, well-being, and quality of life [5,34]. Given the multifaceted potential etiologies, patients with cancer are likely to develop sleep disturbances during some phase of the disease trajectory. Nurses have a pivotal role in minimizing sleep disturbances. They must first be receptive to hearing about them [16]. Primary goals for nursing are to assess for and recognize sleep disturbances, help prevent their development, help determine the etiology, and collaborate with the multidisciplinary team to develop a strategic plan to control or ameliorate this distressing symptom.

References

[1] Savard J, Simard S, Blanchet J, et al. Prevalence, clinical characteristics, and risk factors for insomnia in the context of breast cancer. Sleep 2001;24:583–90.

[2] Kripke DF, Garfinkel L, Wingard DL, et al. Mortality associated with sleep duration and insomnia. Arch Gen Psychiatry 2002;59:131–6.

[3] Clark J, Cunningham M, McMillan S, et al. Sleep-wake disturbances in people with cancer. Part II: evaluating the evidence for clinical decision making. Oncol Nurs Forum 2004;31:747–68.

[4] Silberfarb PM, Hauri PJ, Oxman TE, et al. Assessment of sleep in patients with lung cancer and breast cancer. J Clin Oncol 1993;11:997–1003.

[5] Davidson JR, MacLean AW, Brundage MD, et al. Sleep disturbance in cancer patients. Soc Sci Med 2002;54:1309–21.

[6] Sheely LC. Sleep disturbances in hospitalized patients with cancer. Oncol Nurs Forum 1996;23:109–11.

[7] Hu D, Silberfarb PM. Management of sleep problems in cancer patients. Oncology 1991;5:23–7.

[8] Savard J, Morin C. Insomnia in the context of cancer: a review of a neglected problem. J Clin Oncol 2001; 19:895–908.

[9] Redeker NS, Lev EL, Ruggiero J. Insomnia, fatigue, anxiety, depression and quality of life of cancer patients undergoing chemotherapy. Sch Inq Nurs Pract 2000;14:275–97.

[10] Cannini J, Malcolm R, Peek LA. Treatment of insomnia in cancer patients using muscle relaxation training. J Behav Ther Exp Psychiatry 1983;14:251–6.

[11] Payne S. How is life treating you? Quality of life: a model for cancer care. Prof Nurse 1991;6:531–5.

[12] Silberfarb PM, Hauri PJ, Oxman TE, et al. Insomnia in cancer patients. Soc Sci Med 1985;20:849–50.

[13] Ancoli-Israel S, Moore PJ, Jones V. The relationship between fatigue and sleep in cancer patients: a review. Eur J Cancer Care 2001;10:245–55.

[14] Bovbjerg DH. Circadian disruption and cancer: sleep and immune regulation. Brain Behav Immun 2003; 17(Suppl 1):S48–50.

[15] Malone M, Harris AL, Luscombe DK. Assessment of the impact of cancer on work, recreation, home management and sleep using a general health status measure. J R Soc Med 1994;87:386–9.

[16] Engstrom CA, Strohl RA, Rose L, et al. Sleep alterations in cancer patients. Cancer Nurs 1999;22: 143–8.

[17] Vena C. Sleep-wake patterns in advanced lung and colorectal cancer patients [doctoral dissertation]. Atlanta: Emory University; 2004.

[18] Carskadan MA, Dement WC. Normal human sleep: an overview. In: Kruger MH, Roth T, Dement WC, editors. Principles and practice of sleep medicine. 3rd edition. Philadelphia: WB Saunders; 2000. p. 15–25.

[19] Thomas CD. Insomnia: identification and management. Semin Oncol Nurs 1987;3:263–6.

[20] Owen DC, Parker KP, McGuire DB. Comparison of subjective sleep quality in patients with cancer and healthy subjects. Oncol Nurs Forum 1999;26: 1649–51.

[21] Gupta NE. Snooze blues: women with cancer often suffer from insomnia. Ideas and resources for recovery. MAMM 2001;4:59–60.

[22] Kaye J, Kaye K, Madow L. Sleep patterns in patients with cancer and patients with cardiac disease. J Psychol 1983;114:107–13.

[23] Degner LF, Sloan JA. Symptom distress in newly diagnosed ambulatory cancer patients and as a predictor of survival in lung cancer. J Pain Symptom Manage 1995;10:423–31.

[24] Ginsburg ML, Quirt C, Ginsburg AD, et al. Psychiatric illness and psychosocial concerns of patients with newly diagnosed lung cancer. Can Med Assoc J 1995;152:701–9.

[25] Krech RL, Walsh D. Symptoms of pancreatic cancer. J Pain Symptom Manage 1991;6:360–7.

[26] Kurtz ME, Kurtz JC, Given CW, et al. Loss of physical functioning among patients with cancer. Cancer Pract 1993;1:275–81.

[27] Anderson KO, Getto CJ, Mendoza TR, et al. Fatigue and sleep disturbance in patients with cancer, patients with clinical depression, and community-dwelling adults. J Pain Symptom Manage 2003;25:307–18.

[28] Lamb M. The sleeping patterns of patients with malignant and non-malignant diseases. Cancer Nurs 1982;5:389–96.

[29] Beszterczey A, Lipowski Z. Insomnia in cancer patients. Can Med Assoc J 1977;116:355.

[30] Mills M, Graci GM. Sleep disturbances. In: Yarbro CH, Frogge MH, Goodman M, editors. Cancer symptom management. 3rd edition. Boston: Jones and Bartlett; 2004. p. 111–28.

[31] Couzi RJ, Helzlsouer KJ, Fetting JH. Prevalence of menopausal symptoms among women with a history of breast cancer and attitudes toward estrogen replacement therapy. J Clin Oncol 1995;13:2737–44.

[32] Sateia MD, Silberfarb PM. Sleep in palliative care. In: Doyle D, Hanks GW, MacDonald N, editors. Oxford textbook of palliative medicine. 2nd edition. New York: Oxford University Press; 1998. p. 472–86.

[33] Hirst A, Sloan R. Benzodiazepines and related drugs for insomnia in palliative care. Cochrane Database Syst Rev 2002;4:CD003346.

[34] Vena C, Parker K, Cunningham M, et al. Sleep-wake disturbances in people with cancer. Part I: an overview of sleep, sleep regulation, and effects of disease and treatment. Oncol Nurs Forum 2004;31:735–46.

[35] Mormont MC, Levi F. Circadian system alterations during cancer processes: a review. Int J Cancer 1997; 70:241–7.

[36] Visser MR, Smets EM. Fatigue, depression and quality of life in cancer patients: how are they related? Support Care Cancer 1998;6:101–8.

[37] Moore P, Dimsdale JE. Opioids, sleep, and cancer-related fatigue. Med Hypotheses 2002;58:77–82.

[38] Benca RM, Quintans J. Sleep and host defenses: a review. Sleep 1997;20:1027–37.

[39] Bonnet MH. Effect of sleep disruption on sleep, performance, mood. Sleep 1985;8:11.

[40] Morin CM. Insomnia: psychological assessment and management. New York: Guilford Press; 1993.

[41] Ford DE, Kamerow DB. Epidemiologic study of sleep disturbances and psychiatric disorders. JAMA 1989;262:1479–84.

[42] Hajak G. Insomnia in primary care. Sleep 2000; 23(Suppl 3):S54–63.

[43] Lee K. An overview of sleep and common sleep problems. Am Nephrology Nurse Assoc J 1997;24: 614–25.

[44] Winningham M. How exercise mitigates fatigue: implications for people receiving cancer therapy. In: Carroll-Johnson RM, editor. The biotherapy of cancer. Pittsburgh (PA): Oncology Nursing Society; 1998. p. 16–21.

[45] Sutherland JH, Lockwood GA, Boyd NF. Ratings of the importance of quality of life variables: therapeutic implications for patients with metastatic breast cancer. J Clin Epidemiol 1990;43:661–6.

[46] Morin CM, Ware JC. Sleep and psychopathology. Appl Prev Psychol 1996;5:211–24.

[47] Omne-Ponten M, Holmberg L, Burns T, et al. Determinants of the psycho-social outcome after operation for breast cancer: results of a prospective comparative interview study following mastectomy and breast conservation. Eur J Cancer 1992;28A: 1062–7.

[48] Walsh D, Donnelly S, Rybicki L. The symptoms of advanced cancer: relationship to age, gender, and performance status of 1,000 patients. Support Care Cancer 2000;8:175–9.

[49] Cimprich B. Pretreatment symptom distress in women newly diagnosed with breast cancer. Cancer Nurs 1999;22:185–94.

[50] Ohayon MM, Caulet M, Priest RG, et al. DSM-IV and ICSD-90 insomnia symptoms and sleep dissatisfaction. Br J Psychiatry 1997;171:382–8.

[51] Bliwise DL. Normal aging. In: Kryger MH, Roth T, Dement WC, editors. Principles and practice of sleep medicine. 3rd edition. Philadelphia: WB Saunders; 2000. p. 26–42.

[52] Miaskowski C, Lee K. Pain fatigue, and sleep disturbances in oncology outpatients receiving radiation therapy for bone metastasis: a pilot study. J Pain Symptom Manage 1999;17:320–32.

[53] Dorrepaal KL, Aaronson NK, van Dam FS. Pain experience and pain management among hospitalized cancer patients. Cancer 1989;63:593–8.

[54] Portenoy RK, Miransky J, Thaler HT, et al. Pain in ambulatory patients with lung or colon cancer: prevalence, characteristics, and effect. Cancer 1992; 70:1616–24.

[55] Strang P, Quarner H. Cancer-related pain and its influence on quality of life. Anticancer Res 1990;10: 109–12.

[56] Donovan M, Dilon P, McGuire L. Incidence and characteristics of pain in a sample of medical-surgical inpatients. Pain 1987;30:69–78.

[57] Tamburini M, Selmi S, DeConno F, et al. Semantic descriptors of pain. Pain 1987;29:187–93.

[58] Onen SH, Alloui A, Gross A, et al. The effects of total sleep deprivation, selective sleep interruption and sleep recovery on pain tolerance thresholds in healthy subjects. J Sleep Res 2001;10:35–42.

[59] Corli O, Cozzolino A, Scaricabarozzi I. Nimesulide and diclofenac in the control of cancer-related pain: comparison between oral and rectal administration. Drugs 1993;46(Suppl 1):152–5.

[60] Carrol EN, Fine E, Ruff RL, et al. A four-drug regimen for head and neck cancers. Laryngoscope 1994;104:694–700.

[61] Sjoberg M, Nitescu P, Appelgren L, et al. Long-term intrathecal morphine and bupivacaine in patients with refractory cancer pain. Anesthesiology 1994;80: 284–97.

[62] Cleeland CS, Gonin R, Hatfield AK, et al. Pain and its treatment in outpatients with metastatic cancer. N Engl J Med 1994;330:592–6.

[63] Higginson IJ, Hearn J. A multicenter evaluation of pain control by palliative care teams. J Pain Symptom Manage 1997;14:29–35.

[64] Vainio A, Auvinen A. Prevalence of symptoms among patients with advanced cancer: an international collaborative study. Symptom prevalence group. J Pain Symptom Manage 1996;12:3–10.

[65] Ripamonti C, Zecca E, Brunelli C, et al. Pain experienced by patients hospitalized at the National Cancer Institute of Milan: research project towards a pain-free hospital. Tumori 2000;86:412–8.

[66] Meuser T, Pietruck C, Radbruch L, et al. Symptoms during cancer pain treatment following WHO guidelines: a longitudinal follow-up study of symptom prevalence, severity and etiology. Pain 2001;93: 247–57.

[67] Lawrence CC, Gilbert CJ, Peters WP. Evaluation of symptom distress in a bone marrow transplant outpatient environment. Ann Pharmacother 1996;30: 941–5.

[68] Berger AM, Farr L. The influence of daytime inactivity and nighttime restlessness on cancer-related fatigue. Oncol Nurs Forum 1999;26:1663–71.

[69] Berger AM, Higginbotham P. Correlates of fatigue during and following adjuvant breast cancer chemotherapy: a pilot study. Oncol Nurs Forum 2000;27: 1443–8.

[70] Broeckl JA, Jacobsen PB, Horton J, et al. Characteristics and correlates of fatigue after adjuvant chemotherapy for breast cancer. J Clin Oncol 1998;16: 1689–96.

[71] Belka C, Budach W, Kortman RD, et al. Radiation-induced CNS toxicity-molecular and cellular mechanisms. Br J Cancer 2001;85:1233–9.

[72] Greenberg DB, Gray JL, Mannix CM, et al. Treatment-related fatigue and serum interleukin-1 levels in patients during external beam irradiation for prostate cancer. J Pain Symptom Manage 1993;8: 196–200.

[73] Fortner BV, Septanski EJ, Wang SC, et al. Sleep and quality of life in breast cancer patients. J Pain Symptom Manage 2002;24:471–80.

[74] Carpenter JS, Gautam S, Freedman RR, et al. Circadian rhythm of objectively recorded hot flashes in postmenopausal breast cancer survivors. Menopause 2001;8:181–8.

[75] Mourits MJ, DeVries EG, Willemse PH, et al. Tamoxifen treatment and gynecologic side effects: a review. Obstet Gynecol 2001;97(5 pt 2):855–66.

[76] Polo-Kantola P, Erkkola R, Helenius H, et al. When does estrogen replacement therapy improve sleep quality? Am J Obstet Gynecol 1998;178:1002–9.

[77] Stein KD, Jacobsen PB, Hann DM, et al. Impact of hot flashes on quality of life among postmenopausal women being treated for breast cancer. J Pain Symptom Manage 2000;19:436–45.

[78] Aldrich MS. Sleep medicine. New York: Oxford University Press; 1999.

[79] Ulander K, Grahn G, Sundahl G, et al. Needs and care of patients undergoing subtotal pancreatectomy for cancer. Cancer Nurs 1991;14:27–34.

[80] Topf M, Thompson S. Interactive relationships between hospital patients' noise-induced stress and other stress with sleep. Heart Lung 2001;30:237–43.

[81] Sephton SE, Sapolsky H, Kraemer DS. Diurnal cortisol rhythm as a predictor of breast cancer survival. J Natl Cancer Inst 2000;92:994–9.

[82] Van Cauter E. Endocrine physiology. In: Kryger MH, Roth T, Dement WC, editors. Principles and practice of sleep medicine. 3rd edition. Philadelphia: WB Saunders; 2000. p. 266–78.

[83] Winkelman C. Inactivity and inflammation: selected cytokines as biologic mediators in muscle dysfunction during critical illness. AACN Clin Issues Adv Pract Acute Crit Care 2004;15:74–82.

[84] Klerman EB, Rimmer DW, Dijk D, et al. Nonphotic entrainment of the human circadian pacemaker. Am J Physiol 1998;43:991–6.

[85] Capuron L, Ravaud A, Dantzer R. Early depressive symptoms in cancer patients receiving interleukin-2 and/or interferon alfa-2b therapy. J Clin Oncol 2000; 18:2143–51.

[86] Davidson JR, Waisberg JL, Brundage MD, et al. Nonpharmacologic group treatment of insomnia: a preliminary study with cancer survivors. Psychooncology 2001;10:389–97.

[87] Friedman M, Landsberg R, Pryor S, et al. The occurrence of sleep-disordered breathing among patients with head and neck cancer. Laryngoscope 2001;111(11 Pt 1):1917–9.

[88] Given B, Given C, Azzouz F, et al. Physical functioning of elderly cancer patients prior to diagnosis and following initial treatment. Nurs Res 2001;50: 222–32.

[89] Simon GE, VonKorff M. Prevalence, burden, and

treatment of insomnia in primary care. Am J Psychiatry 1997;154:1417–23.

[90] Derogatis LR, Feldstein M, Morrow G, et al. A survey of psychotropic drug prescriptions in an oncology population. Cancer 1979;44:1919–29.

[91] Bruera E, Fainsinger RL, Schoeller T, et al. Rapid discontinuation of hypnotics in terminal cancer patients: a prospective study. Ann Oncol 1996;7: 85–6.

[92] Hall N. Taking policy action to reduce benzodiazepine use and promote self-care among seniors. J Appl Gerontol 1998;17:318–51.

[93] Holbrook AM, Crowther R, Lotter A, et al. Meta-analysis of benzodiazepine use in the treatment of insomnia. Can Med Assoc J 2000;162:225–33.

[94] Dolan JF. The self-management of sleep interruptions, pain and nausea by adult oncology outpatients: an investigation. Diss Abstr Int B 1984;45:826.

[95] Quesnel C, Savard J, Simard S, et al. Efficacy of cognitive-behavioral therapy for insomnia in women treated for non-metastatic breast cancer. J Consult Clin Psychol 2003;71:189–200.

[96] Berger AM, VonEssen S, Kuhn BR, et al. Adherence, sleep, and fatigue outcomes after adjuvant breast cancer chemotherapy: results of a feasibility intervention study. Oncol Nurs Forum 2003;30:512–22.

[97] Young-McCaughan S, Mays MZ, Arzola SM, et al. Research and commentary: change in exercise tolerance, activity and sleep patterns, and quality of life in patients with cancer participating in a structured exercise program. Oncol Nurs Forum 2003;30: 441–54.

[98] Kim Y, Roscoe JA, Morrow GR. The effects of information and negative affect on severity of side effects from radiation therapy for prostate cancer. Support Care Cancer 2002;10:416–22.

[99] Faithfull S. Patients' experiences following cranial radiotherapy: a study of somnolence syndrome. J Adv Nurs 1991;16:939–46.

[100] Shapiro SL, Bootzin RR, Figueredo AJ, et al. The efficacy of mindfulness-based stress reduction in the treatment of sleep disturbance in women with breast cancer: an exploratory study. J Psychosom Res 2003;54:85–91.

[101] Valdimarsdottir U, Helgason AR, Furst CJ, et al. The unrecognised cost of cancer patients' unrelieved symptoms: a nationwide follow-up of their surviving partners. Br J Cancer 2002;86:1540–5.

[102] McNeil B, Padrick K, Sellman J. I didn't sleep a wink. Am J Nurs 1986;86:26–7.

[103] Kramer M, Kupfer D, Pollak C. When the patterns of sleep go askew. Patient Care 1980;14:122–76.

ELSEVIER
SAUNDERS

Crit Care Nurs Clin N Am 17 (2005) 239–244

CRITICAL CARE
NURSING CLINICS
OF NORTH AMERICA

Sleep and Sedation in the Pediatric Intensive Care Unit

Margaret-Ann Carno, PhD, MBA, RNC, CCRN[a,*], Heidi V. Connolly, MD[b]

[a]University of Rochester School of Nursing, 601 Elmwood Avenue, Box SON, Rochester, NY 14642, USA
[b]Pediatric Critical Care and Sleep Medicine, University of Rochester, 601 Elmwood Avenue, Box 667,
Rochester, NY 14642, USA

Sleep is a basic homeostatic need for the human body. In illness, the need for sleep is even greater. Sleep is an active physiologic process that seems to be a biologic imperative, necessary for maintaining life itself. Specific stages of sleep are integrally related to various bodily functions. For example, rapid eye movement (REM) sleep is necessary for memory consolidation, whereas growth hormone release that occurs during slow wave sleep (SWS) is associated with both somatic growth and various other neuroendocrine functions. Even cortisol release follows a circadian rhythm, peaking in the early hours of the morning shortly before awakening. Sleep is an active process inherently different from the sedated state or from a quiet resting state.

Sleep deprivation has measurable negative consequences. Sleep disruption from either imposed or voluntary sleep restriction and from sleep disorders, such as obstructive sleep apnea, is associated with increased oppositional and inattentive behaviors. Furthermore, sleep deprivation is associated with enhanced perception of chronic pain and worsening of mood disorders, such as depression. These negative consequences of sleep deprivation potentially make providing care for the critically ill child more difficult.

By the very act of providing critical care services, caregivers disrupt necessary sleep. Medications administered to provide adequate analgesia and to help with attaining sufficient cooperation to maintain invasive equipment also interfere with the sleep process. Furthermore, creating an environment in which staff is optimally alert and able to provide complex medical services on short notice is inherently an environment that disrupts sleep for the patient. This article examines what is known about sleep in the pediatric intensive care unit (PICU) and some of the medications administered that interfere with sleep.

What is sleep?

Sleep is a state of disengagement from and unresponsiveness to the environment [1]. It is an active and thought to be restorative process. During this time there are a number of physiologic processes that occur for repair and growth of the human body, such as protein synthesis, growth hormone, and cortisol secretion [2,3]. When sleep is disrupted, negative physiologic (eg, immune), cognitive, and psychologic sequelae occur, thereby disrupting normal human homeostasis and growth [4–6].

There are two categories of sleep: non-REM and REM [1]. Both are needed for the homeostatic effects of sleep. Non-REM sleep is made up of four distinct stages (1–4) with increasing depth of sleep. Non-REM stages 3 and 4 are also called SWS. REM sleep, the stage of sleep in which dreaming occurs, is not broken down into different stages. The pattern of sleep occurs in a predictable fashion. Sleep onset occurs with light sleep (non-REM stages 1 and 2). Most SWS occurs early during the sleep period, whereas most REM sleep occurs during the later part of the sleep period. Cyclic shifts in sleep states occur approximately every 90 minutes throughout the sleep period.

* Corresponding author.
E-mail address: margaret_carno@urmc.rochester.edu
(M.-A. Carno).

Normal sleep in children

Sleep in children follows a characteristic matura-tion pathway [7]. On average infants have a total sleep time of 16 to 18 hours per 24-hour period. In infancy, this sleep occurs throughout the day. As the infant develops, sleep becomes consolidated in the night [7]. A 1-year-old child requires approximately 12 hours of sleep per day that is typically consoli-dated into large sleep periods with one to two daytime naps and a larger period of nighttime sleep. The amount of sleep decreases to 9.5 hours during the adolescent period [7]. Receipt of insufficient quanti-ties of sleep results in negative neurobehavioral con-sequences [6].

Sleep in newborn infants is divided into active and quiet sleep and lacks the electroencephalographic (EEG) features of more mature adult sleep. As the child matures, EEG patterns during sleep also mature. At about 6 months of age scoreable (or adultlike) sleep is present. Of note, delay in the development of EEG sleep patterns to a more adultlike pattern is associated with global developmental delay [8].

Effects of disruption of sleep

Changes in sleep patterns affect the homeostatic processes of the body. Sleep disruption effects the immune system, hypothalamic-pituitary axis, psycho-logic, and cognitive functioning [5,6]. It is known that SWS inhibits the hypothalamic-pituitary axis and cortisol secretion [3]. Sleep restriction causes in-creased cortisol secretion and changes in secretion pattern [4]. In relation to the immune system, Dinges and coworkers [6] examined healthy adults who underwent sleep deprivation. Acute sleep loss pro-duced fatigue, cognitive performance failure, and an increase in total white blood cell count. The change in white blood cell count was characterized by a marked increase in monocytes, supporting a potential key role in immune response to sleep loss. Similar findings were reported from a study of the effects of 48-hour sleep deprivation on healthy adult men [9].

Sleep in children in the pediatric intensive care unit

The literature of sleep in the PICU is scarce. Only four studies examining sleep in the PICU were uncovered during a literature search. In 1996, Corser [10] published her work examining sleep in 1- to 2-year-old children who had been admitted to the

PICU. Twelve children (six boys) were enrolled in the study with an age range of 23.33 ± 6.08 (SD) months. The children had an average Pediatric Risk Mortality Score of 5.08 ± 4.19 and an average length of stay of 12.17 ± 27.95 days. The variables included sleep state (as noted by observation); medications administered; caregiver disruptions; and noise and light levels. The Patient Sleep Behavior Observation Tool was used to assess sleep states. This tool, developed in 1968 by Echols, describes four levels of cortical vigilance [10]. Each child was observed throughout the night for 12 hours and every 5 min-utes sleep state and other information were noted. The mean total sleep time was 438.83 ± 166.98 (SD) minutes with a range of 135 to 645 minutes [10]. This corresponds to 7.3 ± 2.78 hours (range 2.25–10.75 hours), a marked decrease for the amount of sleep required in this age group. The longest sleep period was 128.74 ± 46.76 minutes (range 40–180). The children awoke 9.03 ± 4.4 (range 3–16) times during the night. There were negative correlations between sleep state, light levels, noise levels, care-giver activities, and pain level [10]. There was a positive correlation between total sleep time and the amount of benzodiazepine given [10].

A study examining sleep in the PICU with an older subject group was published in 1997 [11]. This study also used the Patient Sleep Behavior Observa-tion Tool to stage sleep by caregiver observations, which according to the authors measures the four cortical states of (1) awake; (2) drowsy; (3) para-doxical sleep (REM); and (4) orthodoxical sleep (non-REM) [11]. Noise and light levels along with caregiver activities were also measured. The children were observed from 8:00 PM until 6:00 AM on one night and information was collected at 5-minute time intervals. Parental presence was also noted [11]. Nine children (four girls) with an age of 4.7 ± 3.5 years (range 15 months–10.5 years) were enrolled in the study. Pediatric Risk Mortality Score was calculated but not reported. The authors state that all the children had either a low or moderate severity of illness; length of stay was not reported [11]. The children slept on average 4.7 ± 0.49 (SD) hours with a mean sleep length of 27.6 ± 25.85 (SD) minutes. The average number of awakenings (either caused by caregiver contact or spontaneous) was 9.8 ± 2.48 (SD) (range 6–14). Noise levels were reported with a mean of 55.1 ± 6.82 (SD) dB(A) (range 4–95 dB[A]) and an average light level of 23.4 ± 22.85 (SD) foot-candle (range 5–140 ft-candle). The number of caregiver contacts was 10.8 ± 4.18 (SD) with a mean duration of 14.1 ± 9.84 minutes [11]. Parents were present 28.1% ± 38.29% (SD) of the time during the study period. For purpose of analysis the authors collapsed the Patient Sleep Behavior Observation Tool categories to awake or sleeping. Using probit analysis, noise level, light level, and contact with staff were significant predictors of sleep [11]. The amount of sleep achieved by the subjects is much less than what was anticipated in this age group.

Using a semistructured interview technique children were asked about their experiences in the PICU [12]. Thirty-eight children, 4 to 16 years of age, were enrolled in the study. Sixty-six percent of the children remembered the PICU and that 16% complained of being unable to sleep because of the noise or discomfort [12].

Using an objective measure of sleep (polysomnography) Carno and coworkers [13] reported a pilot study examining the patterns of sleep in children undergoing neuromuscular blockade and sedation, a common therapy in the PICU. Neuromuscular blockade was an exclusion criterion in the Corser [10] and Cureton-Lane and Fontaine studies [11]. Two children, both 3 years of age, were enrolled in the study after surgical repair of subglottic stenosis using a single-stage laryngotracheoplasty. Polysomnography recordings were continuous over a 96-hour period for each child, measuring sleep during the day to nighttime. Subject 1 received continuous opioid infusion along with neuromuscular blockade. Subject 2 received continuous opioid infusion and supplemental doses administered based on nurse assessment. This subject received lorazepam and chloral hydrate to achieve sufficient sedation as determined by the bedside nurses' assessment. There was no attempt to influence the type or amount of medication administered (either sedation or neuromuscular blockade) by the research team [13].

Adult data have shown that in critically ill patients' sleep occurs throughout the day and is not consolidated to the nighttime [14]. As expected, sleep occurred throughout a 24-hour period. A marked shift to lighter stages of sleep was noted in each subject. Subject 1 spent 50% of the total time in stage 1 sleep and 41% of the total recording time in stage 2 sleep [13]. Because eye movements are needed to determine REM sleep or wakefulness and eye movements are lost with neuromuscular blockade, the study team described this stage as non-REM sleep. Subject 1 spent 9% of the total recording time in non-REM sleep [13]. Subject 2 spent 11% of the recording time in stage 1 sleep, 63% in stage 2, 4% in stage 3, and 22% in non-REM sleep. For both subjects, the percentage of total sleep time spent at specific stages was markedly different than what would be expected for a normal 3-year-old child but because of the small

sample size, statistical evaluation could not be performed [13]. Notably, SWS was diminished in both subjects.

These studies show that sleep is disrupted in the PICU in a number of children across diagnoses. Interventions in improving sleep in the PICU are needed.

Nonpharmacologic methods to improve sleep in the pediatric intensive care unit

There is a lack of published data on attempts to improve sleep patterns in the PICU. In the adult literature there have been attempts to improve sleep using nonpharmacologic methods (including imagery and relaxation and changes in the environment) with varying degrees of success [15–18]. Implementing changes in the environment (such as "quiet hour," and staff behavior modification decreasing noise and light levels during the night time) have all met with difficulties in implementation [15–17].

Sleep versus sedation

The purpose of sedation in the PICU is to decrease anxiety, agitation, maintenance of invasive lines, and to facilitate mechanical ventilation [19]. Agitation and anxiety can occur from a number of factors including fear of the unknown, inability to understand what is happening, and being unable to communicate needs [19]. Sedation has been shown to improve the ability of the patient to tolerate ICU care. Although many commonly used analgesics also provide sedation (eg, narcotics), this is not uniformly true (eg, acetaminophen, ketorolac tromethamine). Similarly, many sedatives commonly used in the PICU do not provide analgesia (eg, benzodiazepines, propofol). Sedation is not synonymous with analgesia (removal of pain) [19].

When a patient (or child) is sedated they look comfortable and even asleep, but this sedative or chemical sleep is not thought to have the same restorative effect for physiologic processes that does natural sleep. Most, if not all, medications used in the PICU affect the normal sleep process [20]. Both the administration and withdrawal of a medication can affect sleep negatively.

When assessing a patient at the bedside, priority should be directed at providing adequate analgesia. Pain is known to disrupt sleep and cause agitation. Ineffective pain relief has been associated with poor outcomes. In a landmark study published in 1987 and follow-up study in 1992 Anand and coworkers

[21,22] demonstrated that infants undergoing a patent ductus arteriosus ligation had decreased morbidity and improved survivorship when they received narcotic analgesia in comparison with a group who did not. Frequent, accurate assessment for pain is the first step in providing effective sedation. Some older children hide pain by closing their eyes and not moving, whereas others grimace and cry. Relaxation predictably occurs with adequate pain control. Medications used for analgesia can also affect sleep patterns. Proper analgesia is essential before sedatives can be administered.

Effects on sleep of commonly administered medications in the pediatric intensive care unit for analgesia and sedation

Medications for analgesia

Most medications administered in the PICU for analgesia belong to the opiate family. There are naturally derived opiates (morphine) and semisynthetic (fentanyl). All increase total sleep time but result in more disrupted sleep. There is also a decrease in REM sleep with opiates [20]. Although the child looks asleep, the sleep is not restorative or restful. Effective pain relief may still help the child fall asleep even if the sleep obtained is disruptive.

Sedative medications

Benzodiazepines are commonly used for sedation in the PICU. This includes diazepam, midazolam, and lorazepam. This class of drugs increases total sleep time and stage 2 sleep, while decreasing stage 1 and SWS [20]. Unfortunately, the shorter-acting benzodiazepines can cause sleep fragmentation in the later portion of the night (as they wear off) decreasing the amount of restful sleep [20].

Measuring sedation in the pediatric intensive care unit

Sedation scores
The ability to determine the level of sedation in the pediatric population is a challenge for the bedside nurse. There are a number of different tools to assist the bedside nurse. The three most frequently used in the pediatric population are (1) the Ramsey Scale, (2) the Comfort Scale, and (3) the University of Michigan Sedation Scale (UMSS) [23,24]. The Ramsey Scale was developed in the early 1970s and validated using an adult population and measures

anxiety level from agitated and anxious to no response on a scale from 1 to 6 [23]. The higher the score the more sedate the patient [23].

The Comfort Scale was developed initially in the 1960s and revised in the 1980s specifically for the pediatric ICU population by Ambuel [23]. The scale measures eight domains that include alertness, agitation level, respiratory response, physical movement, blood pressure, heart rate, muscle tone, and facial tone, with five sublevels for each domain [23]. The lower the score the more sedate the child. The reported Cronbach's alpha is 0.9 and a correlation coefficient of 0.75 to 0.84 [23].

The UMSS was designed for use in determining level of sedation for procedures in a pediatric population but also has been used in the PICU [24]. The scale has five levels from awake to unarousable with a higher score indicative of deeper sedation [24]. The validation data for the PICU are lacking but the reported kappa score of agreement is 0.59 to 0.84 in children undergoing sedation during invasive procedures [24].

BIS monitoring
The bispectral (BIS) index monitor is a measure of EEG frequency and as such a measure of the depth of anesthesia and sedation [25]. The index is a scale from 0 to 100 and the monitor measures the degree of coherence among different frequencies of the electrocephalograph [25]. It was first developed in EEG recordings of healthy adults for determining level of anesthesia in the operating room [26]. Although most of the data using the BIS monitor are in the adult population, there have been a few studies examining the use of the BIS monitor in the pediatric population.

McDermott and coworkers [26] examined 86 children ($\leq$12 years of age) who were undergoing elective diagnostic or therapeutic procedures that involved conscious or deep sedation and compared the BIS monitor results with a validated pediatric sedation scale (UMSS). A variety of sedatives were used during the study. UMSS sedation score was closely correlated with the BIS score ($P < .0001$). The authors conclude that the BIS is a valid monitor of sedation level in the pediatric population. The BIS monitor has also been compared with the Ramsey Scale (modified for pediatric patients) and the Comfort score with a small to moderate correlation to both (Ramsey $r^2 = 0.12$ $P < .0001$; Comfort $r^2 = 0.25$ $P < .0001$) [27,28].

BIS monitoring and sleep states
There have been attempts to use BIS monitoring to predict and monitor physiologic sleep states.

Sleigh and coworkers [25] examined BIS monitoring in five adults sleeping in their own home. None of the subjects were receiving any medications that would affect sleep. Numerical BIS scores varied with specific sleep states. Awake state had a BIS level of 92 ± 3; light sleep had a reported BIS level of 81 ± 9; SWS (or deep sleep) had a BIS level of 59 ± 10; and REM sleep resulted in a BIS score of 83 ± 6 [25]. There was overlap between BIS levels during different sleep states, in particular awake, light sleep, and REM. Studies assessing the correlation between BIS score and EEG-staged sleep in the ICU is lacking.

Nieuwenhuijs and coworkers [29] also examined the role of BIS monitoring for sleep states in 10 adult subjects during evaluation for mild obstructive sleep apnea. Although the BIS levels did decrease with depth of sleep, they found a large overlap in BIS values at each sleep stage. Light sleep had a BIS value of 40 to 80, SWS values were 35 to 70, and REM sleep had BIS values of 40 to 60 [29]. The authors of this paper conclude that BIS is not an adequate measure to assess sleep state.

Summary

Sleep is a restorative process that maintains homeostatic processes in the human body. Sleep in the PICU is disturbed and the physiologic and psychologic ramifications are yet to be elucidated. Further research in this area needs to be conducted. Based on the knowledge that sleep is important for maintenance of proper immune function, hypothalamic-pituitary axis, and growth, it is likely that sleep disruption resulting from hospitalization in the PICU negatively impacts important bodily functions. Nursing has a unique role as the bedside caregiver in moving this research forward and applying the findings to the bedside.

References

[1] Carskadon M, Dement W. Normal human sleep. In: Kryger M, Roth T, Dement W, editors. Principles and practice of sleep medicine. 3rd edition. Philadelphia: WB Saunders; 2000. p. 15–25.

[2] Redwine L, Hauger RL, Gillin JC, et al. Effects of sleep and sleep deprivation on interleukin-6, growth hormone, cortisol, and melatonin levels in humans. J Clin Endocrinol Metab 2000;85:3597–603.

[3] Vgontzas AN, Chrousos GP. Sleep, the hypothalamic-pituitary-adrenal axis, and cytokines: multiple inter-

[4] Vgontzas AN, Zoumakis E, Bixler EO, et al. Adverse effects of modest sleep restriction on sleepiness, performance, and inflammatory cytokines. J Clin Endocrinol Metab 2004;89:2119–26.

[5] Steiger A. Sleep and the hypothalamo-pituitary-adrenocortical system. Sleep Med Rev 2002;6:125–38.

[6] Dinges D, Douglas S, Zaugg L, et al. Leukocytosis and natural killer cell function parallel neurobehavioral fatigue induced by 64 hours of sleep deprivation. J Clin Invest 1994;93:1930–9.

[7] Carno M, Hoffman LA, Carcillo JA, et al. Developmental stages of sleep from birth to adolescence, common childhood sleep disorders: overview and nursing implications. J Pediatr Nurs 2003;18:274–83.

[8] Scher MS. Neurophysiological assessment of brain function and maturation: a measure of brain adaptation in high risk infants. Pediatr Neurol 1997;16:191–8.

[9] Ozturk L, Pelin Z, Karadeniz D, et al. Effects of 48 hours of sleep deprivation on human immune profile. Sleep Res Online 1999;2:107–11.

[10] Corser N. Sleep of 1 and 2 year old children in intensive care. Issues Compr Pediatr Nurs 1996;19:17–31.

[11] Cureton-Lane RA, Fontaine DK. Sleep in the pediatric ICU: an empirical investigation. Am J Crit Care 1997; 6:56–63.

[12] Playfor S, Thomas D, Choonara I. Recollection of children following intensive care. Arch Dis Child 2000;83:445–8.

[13] Carno MA, Hoffman LA, Henker R, et al. Sleep monitoring in children during neuromuscular blockade in the pediatric intensive care unit: a pilot study. Pediatr Crit Care Med 2004;5:224–9.

[14] Cooper A, Thornley K, Young B, et al. Sleep in critically ill patients requiring mechanical ventilation. Chest 2000;117:809–18.

[15] Kahn DM, Cook TE, Carlisle CC, et al. Identification and modification of environmental noise in an ICU setting. Chest 1998;114:535–40.

[16] Walder B, Francioli D, Meyer JJ, et al. Effects of guidelines implementation in a surgical intensive care unit to control nighttime light and noise levels. Crit Care Med 2000;28:2242–7.

[17] Olson DM, Borel CO, Laskowitz DT, et al. Quiet time: a nursing intervention to promote sleep in neurocritical care units. Am J Crit Care 2001;10:74–8.

[18] Richardson S. Effects of relaxation and imagery on the sleep of critically ill adults. DCCN: Dimensions of Critical Care Nursing 2003;22:182–90.

[19] American College of Critical Care Medicine of the Society of Critical Care Medicine, American Society of Health-System Pharmacists, American College of Chest Physicians. Clinical practice guidelines for the sustained use of sedatives and analgesics in the critically ill adult. Am J Health Syst Pharm 2000;59:150–78.

[20] Obermeyer WH, Benca RM. Effects of drugs on sleep. Neurol Clin 1996;14:827–40.

[21] Anand KJS, Sippell WG, Aynsley-Green A. Random-

ized trial of fentanyl anaesthesia in preterm babies undergoing surgery: effects on the stress response. Lancet 1987;1:62–6.

[22] Anand KJ, Hickey PR. Halothane-morphine compared with high does sufentanil for anesthesia and postoperative analgesia in neonatal cardiac surgery. N Engl J Med 1992;326:55–6.

[23] De Jonghe B, Cook D, Appere-De-Vecchi C, et al. Using and understanding sedation scoring systems: a systematic review. Intensive Care Med 2000;26:275–85.

[24] Malviya S, Voepel-Lewis T, Tait AR, et al. Depth of sedation in children undergoing computed tomography: validity and reliability of the University of Michigan Sedation Scale (UMSS). Br J Anaesth 2001;88:241–5.

[25] Sleigh JW, Andrzejowski J, Steyn-Ross A, et al. The bispectral index: a measure of sleep? Anesth Analg 1999;88:659–61.

[26] McDermott NB, VanSickle T, Motas D, et al. Validation of the bispectral index monitor during conscious and deep sedation in children. Anesth Analg 2003;97:39–43.

[27] Berkenbosch JW, Fichter CR, Tobias JD. The correlation of the Bispectral Index Monitor with clinical sedation scores during mechanical ventilation in the pediatric intensive care unit. Anesth Analg 2002;94:506–11.

[28] Courtman SP, Wardurgh A, Petros AJ. Comparison of the bispectral index monitor with the Comfort score in assessing level of sedation of critically ill children. Intensive Care Med 2003;29:2239–46.

[29] Nieuwenhuijs D, Coleman EL, Douglas NJ, et al. Bispectral index values and spectral edge frequency at different stages of physiologic sleep. Anesth Analg 2002;94:125–9.

ELSEVIER
SAUNDERS

CRITICAL CARE
NURSING CLINICS
OF NORTH AMERICA

Crit Care Nurs Clin N Am 17 (2005) 245–250

The Effects of Liver and Renal Dysfunction on the Pharmacokinetics of Sedatives and Analgesics in the Critically Ill Patient

Dinesh Yogaratnam, PharmD*, Melissa A. Miller, PharmD, Brian S. Smith, PharmD, BCPS

Department of Pharmacy, University of Massachusetts Memorial Medical Center, Memorial Campus, 119 Belmont Street, Worcester, MA 01605, USA

Sedative and analgesic drugs are often used in the ICU to help achieve the best possible level of comfort and safety for critically ill patients. Pain, anxiety, and agitation can complicate therapeutic and diagnostic procedures, increase the risk of patient self-extubation, and make nursing care significantly more difficult [1]. Numerous factors can contribute to the discomfort of critically ill patients, including mechanical ventilation and invasive procedures. In addition to improving patient tolerance of these interventions, sedation and analgesia may improve morbidity by reducing stress-related inflammation and pulmonary complications [2].

Patients in the ICU can display a wide range of organ dysfunctions. Hepatic dysfunction may be seen in up to half of all critically ill patients, and the incidence of acute renal failure in this population may range between 7% and 23% [3,4]. Alterations in hepatic and renal function can significantly alter the pharmacokinetics (PK) of drugs, which may result in adverse outcomes. Patients with renal or hepatic failure, for example, may experience prolonged exposure to sedative agents, resulting in extra days of mechanical ventilation. This, in turn, increases the risk of developing ventilator-associated pneumonia and lung injury, lengthens the course of hospitalization, and raises the costs of patient care. Being familiar with the principles that govern PK in

critically ill patients can help minimize unintended consequences of sedative and analgesic drug therapy. This article reviews PK and pharmacodynamic (PD) parameters of sedative and opioid analgesic drugs in critically ill patients with hepatic or renal dysfunction.

The liver

The liver has a wide range of functions. It plays a major role in glucose storage and regulation, and it is responsible for the production of clotting factors, cholesterol, and circulating plasma proteins, such as albumin. In addition, the liver is the primary organ involved in the metabolism of drugs and removal of toxic substances from the systemic circulation. Liver dysfunction can profoundly influence the PK of drugs by altering bioavailability, apparent volume of distribution, and clearance [5–7]. These changes, in turn, can affect the pharmacologic duration and potency of sedative and analgesic drugs. The PK parameters for some common sedatives and opioids, as measured in healthy subjects, are shown in Tables 1 and 2.

Bioavailability

Bioavailability is the amount of administered drug that is available to the systemic circulation. Definitions of this and other common PK terms are listed in

---

* Corresponding author.
E-mail address: yogaratd@ummhc.org (D. Yogaratnam).

Table 1
Pharmacokinetics of sedative agents

Drug	Metabolic substrate	Significant metabolite	E	PB (%)	$t\frac{1}{2}$ (h)	Vd (L/kg)
Lorazepam	Glucuronyltransferase	None	Low	91	12	1.3
Diazepam	CYP 2C19	Desmethyldiazepam Oxazepam	Low	99	19–54	1.1
Midazolam	CYP 3A4	α-Hydroxymidazolam	Intermediate	95	1.8–6.4	1–2.5
Propofol	Glucuronyltransferase	None	High	98	1.5–12.4	60

Abbreviations: E, hepatic extraction ratio; PB, protein binding; $t\frac{1}{2}$ (h), elimination half-life expressed in hours; Vd (L/kg), apparent volume of distribution expressed in liters per kilogram.

Box 1. The oral bioavailability of most drugs is generally less than 100% and can vary widely depending on the molecular characteristics of the drug. Drugs administered orally are absorbed through the lining of the small intestine whereby they enter enterohepatic circulation. Before entering systemic circulation, the drug passes through the liver and is exposed to hepatic metabolism. This process is often referred to as the "first-pass effect." When the liver has a compromised ability to metabolize drugs, the first-pass effect can be significantly diminished. For orally administered drugs that are highly sensitive to first-pass metabolism, this may render a substantial increase in systemic bioavailability. In a study involving seven patients with a history of alcoholic cirrhosis and hepatic encephalopathy, the oral bioavailability of a single dose of morphine was found to be more than twice as high as healthy controls [8]. Similarly, the systemic bioavailability of orally administered midazolam has been shown to be significantly larger in patients with cirrhosis as compared with healthy controls [9]. Most sedatives and analgesics in the ICU, however, are given by the intravenous route. Drugs administered intravenously are not subjected to first-pass metabolism and are 100% bioavailable. Other PK parameters besides bioavailability, however, can be altered in critically ill patients with liver disease.

Distribution

Volume of distribution is a relative term, expressed in liters, that describes the degree to which a drug distributes throughout the body. Drugs that are hydrophilic (water-soluble) or highly protein bound have relatively small volumes of distribution, whereas drugs that are lipophilic (lipid-soluble) or not significantly protein bound have relatively large volumes of distribution. Volume of distribution is directly proportional to half-life, and increases in volume of distribution can result in a prolonged therapeutic effect for certain sedative and analgesic drugs.

Patients with severe chronic liver disease, like alcoholic cirrhosis, often display increases in volume of distribution as a result of decreased circulating plasma proteins. Furthermore, critically ill patients often have reduced albumin because of malnutrition or acute illness [10]. Plasma proteins, such as albumin and α1-acid glycoprotein, serve as the primary source of oncotic pressure within the vascular space. Decreases in oncotic pressure may result in fluid shifting out of the intravascular space, which may increase the volume of distribution of hydrophilic drugs. Low serum albumin has been shown to lead to prolonged sedation with midazolam in critically ill patients with renal failure [11]. This effect was shown to be related to an increase in midazolam's

Table 2
Pharmacokinetics of opioid agents

Drug	Metabolic substrate	Significant metabolite	E	PB (%)	$t\frac{1}{2}$ (h)	Vd (L/kg)
Morphine	Glucuronyltransferase	m-3-Glucuronide m-6-Glucuronide	High	36	1.5–4.5	1–4
Fentanyl	CYP 3A4	None	High	84	3.65	3.2–4
Methadone	CYP 3A4	None	Low	89	23	3.6
Hydromorphone	Glucuronyltransferase	hm-6-Glucuronide	Intermediate	71	2.65	1.22

Abbreviations: E, hepatic extraction ratio; hm-6-glucuronide, hydromorphone-6-glucoronide; m-3-glucoronide, morphine-3-glucoronide; m-6-glucuronide, morphine-6-glucoronide; PB, protein binding; $t\frac{1}{2}$ (h), elimination half-life expressed in hours; Vd (L/kg), apparent volume of distribution expressed in liters per kilogram.

Box 1. Pharmacokinetic terms and definitions

Absorption: Process by which a drug enters the systemic circulation

Bioavailability: Fraction of the dose of a drug that reaches the systemic circulation

Clearance: Volume of fluid (usually blood or plasma) that is cleared of drug per unit time

Distribution: Movement of drug between body compartments (eg, between blood vessels and peripheral tissues)

Elimination: Removal of drug from the body through excretion or metabolism

Extraction ratio: Fraction of the drug presented to an eliminating organ that is cleared after a single pass

Half-life: Length of time necessary to reduce the concentration of a drug by 50%

Metabolism: Removal of drug from the body by biotransformation by enzymatic or conjugation reactions

Pharmacokinetics: Effect of the body on the drug (absorption, distribution, metabolism, elimination)

Pharmacodynamics: Effect of the drug on the body (dose-response relationship)

Steady state: Equilibrium condition reached when the rate of administration of a drug equals the rate of elimination

Volume of distribution: Apparent volume in the body in which the drug is dissolved

volume of distribution with a subsequent reduction in its clearance.

Metabolism and clearance

Liver dysfunction can affect the metabolism of drugs by a variety of mechanisms. Reductions in functional hepatic blood flow, decreases in protein binding, and damage to liver cells can reduce the metabolism and clearance of drugs from the plasma.

Cellular metabolism

The predominant hepatic mechanisms involved in the metabolism of sedatives and analgesics include cytochrome P-450 enzyme reactions (phase I metabolism) and conjugation reactions (phase II metabolism). These processes result in the biotransformation of drugs into water-soluble metabolites that can be eliminated through the kidneys or bile. Metabolites can be inactive, possess some degree of pharmacologic activity, or be toxic. Most active metabolites are generally less potent than their parent compound, but they can result in enhanced or prolonged pharmacologic activity if their elimination is retarded. A description of the metabolic by-products of common ICU sedatives and opioids are listed in Tables 1 and 2.

Clearance and blood flow

Clearance is a term used to describe the volume of fluid that is completely cleared of a substance per unit of time. The clearance of sedative and analgesic drugs from the serum is largely dependent on the extent to which the liver can metabolize these agents. Hepatic clearance is the product of the hepatic extraction ratio and hepatic blood flow. The hepatic extraction ratio is the fraction of drug that is removed from circulation after one pass through the liver. With respect to hepatic clearance, drugs with a high extraction ratio (>70%) are significantly affected by changes in hepatic blood flow and less affected by changes in hepatic function. Conversely, drugs with a low extraction ratio (<30%) are much more sensitive to changes in hepatic function and less sensitive to changes in hepatic blood flow [5–7]. Fentanyl is a synthetic opioid analgesic with a high extraction ratio. The PK of intravenous fentanyl has previously been shown to be unaffected in surgical patients with cirrhosis [12]. The authors attributed this lack of effect to the relatively preserved hepatic blood flow observed in the patients.

Clearance and protein binding

Highly protein-bound drugs exist in a state of equilibrium between unbound and bound drug. Because only the unbound (free) form of the drug is pharmacologically active, decreased plasma proteins can lead to an increase in the amount of drug available at the site of action. Protein binding can have a significant impact on the distribution (discussed previously) and metabolism of sedative and analgesic drugs. The plasma protein binding characteristics of a drug can be classified as either nonrestrictive or restrictive. Drugs that display nonrestrictive protein binding are easily dissociated from their carrier proteins, and are readily available for hepatic metabolism [5]. The extent of protein binding for nonrestrictive drugs does not influence the hepatic extraction ratio. For drugs that display restrictive protein binding, only the free, unbound fraction of the drug is available for hepatic metabolism. A decrease in circulating plasma proteins increases the free-fraction of the drug and increases the hepatic extraction ratio. For restrictive drugs, however, an increased fraction of unbound drug also results in a higher concentration of drug that is available for therapeutic action.

Estimates of liver function

Assessing hepatic function in the critically ill can be challenging. Although creatinine clearance is a generally well-accepted indicator of renal function, there is no hepatic correlate that accurately reflects liver function. To help clinicians objectively assess liver function, a number of scoring systems have been developed. These scoring systems take laboratory data (bilirubin, albumin, prothrombin time), clinical features (ascites, encephalopathy, nutrition status), patient history (alcohol abuse), and patient status (hospitalized or ambulatory) into account to assess objectively the degree of hepatic impairment. Examples of such scoring systems include the Child's Score, Child's Score with Pugh's Modification, and the Model for End Stage Liver Disease Score [13–15]. Although these scoring systems are useful in assessing the severity of liver disease and predicting mortality, they have not been validated as drug dosing tools.

The kidneys

The kidneys are responsible for the elimination of many drugs and their metabolites. There are three major mechanisms involved in the renal clearance of drugs: (1) glomerular filtration, (2) tubular secretion, and (3) reabsorption. Of these, glomerular filtration is primarily responsible for the elimination of most drugs and their metabolites.

Glomerular filtration is a passive process. Water-soluble molecules and drugs of small molecular size are filtered more easily than large or protein-bound drugs. As drugs and metabolites pass through the kidneys, they are removed by glomerular filtration and eliminated through the urine.

Effect of renal pathology on drug clearance

The PK and PD of drugs used in critically ill patients are often difficult to predict because of the dynamic physiologic changes that occur in this patient population. Studies of the effects of renal failure on drug PK in critically ill patients are very limited [16]. Most available data are on healthy populations or in patients with chronic renal failure. It is important for clinicians to have a sound understanding of PK and PD principles and to know how to apply these principles to individualize therapy for a critically ill patient. The following discussion focuses on the effects of renal failure on the distribution, metabolism, and elimination of sedatives and analgesics in critically ill patients.

Distribution

Alterations in protein binding can have a profound affect on a drug's volume of distribution. In a related manner, the accumulation of fluid during renal failure can also have an impact on the extent of drug distribution throughout the body. As fluid accumulates, water-soluble drugs are able to diffuse with excess fluid into the extravascular space. This results in a reduced concentration of drug within the intravascular space that is available for metabolism and elimination, which reduces drug clearance. In a related phenomenon, alterations in fluid status can alter the concentration of drug that is presented to the pharmacologic site of action, resulting in a diminished dose-response relationship. Although changes in fluid status are often difficult to predict in critically ill patients with renal dysfunction, clinicians should be aware that sudden fluid shifts, like what may occur following a hemodialysis session, may impart a significant change in the PK and PD of sedative and analgesic agents.

Metabolism

The kidneys are known to have active drug metabolizing systems, and changes to renal and hepatic drug metabolism have been noted in patients with renal failure [17–20]. The clinical significance of these effects on sedatives and analgesics in critically ill patients with renal disease remains to be determined. Careful drug dosing and monitoring is essential to ensure drug therapy is achieving desired pharmacologic effects without causing adverse events.

Elimination

Determining drug elimination in the critically ill patient population is challenging for many reasons. Most PK studies in renally or hepatically impaired patients are usually performed in stable patients with chronic disease effecting only one organ system. It is difficult to apply these data to unstable, critically ill patients with multiple organ dysfunction. In addition, renal drug clearance in critically ill patients can be influenced by a number of comorbidities, including liver failure, hemodynamic instability, and malnutrition.

Reductions in the glomerular filtration rate leading to renal failure may significantly reduce the elimination of drugs and drug metabolites that are primarily eliminated by filtration. The active metabolites of morphine (morphine-3-glucuronide and morphine-6-glucuronide) and midazolam (glucuronidated α-hydroxymidazolam) have been shown to accumulate in critically ill patients with renal failure [21,22]. When using these medications in this patient population, clinicians should consider using alternative agents or empirically reduce the dose. The glucuronide metabolite of lorazepam has also been shown to accumulate in patients with renal failure, but this is of no clinical significance because the metabolite is neither active nor toxic at high concentrations [23].

Estimates of renal clearance

Assessing renal function in critically ill patients is a challenging but important step in appropriately dosing drugs that are removed by the kidneys. For renally eliminated drugs, the rate of elimination is often directly proportional to the glomerular filtration rate. The creatinine clearance is the most frequently used estimate of glomerular filtration rate, and this value can be measured by collecting 24-hour urine creatinine production or estimated by using calculations based on serum creatinine or other laboratory measures. There are many equations that can be used to estimate creatinine clearance, but the one that is most often used to guide drug dosing is the Cockroft and Gault equation [24–28]. It is important to stress that there are many conditions and situations in critically ill patients that alter the accuracy of any of these methods, including the Cockroft and Gault equation. For example, in renally impaired patients who also have cirrhosis, creatinine-based estimates of renal function have been shown to overestimate glomerular filtration rate to varying degrees [29].

Summary

There are many factors besides organ dysfunction that can alter the PK and PD of drug therapy. In ICU patients with hepatic or renal dysfunction, drug disposition can be influenced by the presence of comorbid conditions, drug interactions, and the use of hemodialysis. To ensure optimal dosing of sedatives and analgesics, and to promote positive therapeutic outcomes, regular and repeated clinical assessments need to be performed [30,31]. There are several bedside assessment tools that are used to assess the adequacy of sedation, including the Richmond Agitation-Sedation Scale, the Sedation-Agitation Scale, the Motor Activity Assessment Scale, and the Ramsey Sedation Scale [31]. The bispectral index, which is a statistically derived variable of the electroencephalogram, is an objective measure of sedation that has undergone limited validity testing in the ICU [32]. Regardless of the sedation scale that is used, it is important that patients in the ICU are monitored regularly. Regular assessment of sedation and pain control minimizes the risks of oversedation and undersedation and reduces the number of unnecessary procedures that are performed to exclude other reasons for unresponsiveness [2,30].

The presence of renal or hepatic dysfunction in the critically ill patient can significantly alter the PK and PD of sedatives and opioid analgesics. By anticipating these changes and routinely assessing the response to therapy, health care providers can offer effective treatment regimens that minimize adverse events.

References

[1] Atkins PM, Mion LC, Mendelson W, et al. Characteristics and outcomes of patients who self-extubate from ventilatory support: a case-control study. Chest 1997; 112:1317–23.

[2] Walder B, Tramer MR. Analgesia and sedation in critically ill patients. Swiss Med Wkly 2004;134:333–46.

[3] Power BM, Forbes AM, van Heerden PV, et al. Pharmacokinetics of drugs used in critically ill adults. Clin Pharmacokinet 1998;34:25–56.

[4] al-Khafaji A, Corwin HL. Acute renal failure and dialysis in the chronically critically ill patient. Clin Chest Med 2001;22:165–74.

[5] Howden CW, Birnie GG, Brodie MJ. Drug metabolism in liver disease. Pharmacol Ther 1989;40:439–74.

[6] Rodighiero V. Effects of liver disease on pharmacokinetics: an update. Clin Pharmacokinet 1999;37: 399–431.

[7] Tegeder I, Lotsch J, Geisslinger G. Pharmacokinetics

of opioids in liver disease. Clin Pharmacokinet 1999; 37:17–40.

[8] Hasselstrom J, Eriksson S, Persson A, et al. The metabolism and bioavailability of morphine in patients with severe liver cirrhosis. Br J Clin Pharmacol 1990; 29:289–97.

[9] Pentikainen PJ, Valisalmi L, Himberg JJ, et al. Pharmacokinetics of midazolam following intravenous and oral administration in patients with chronic liver disease and in healthy subjects. J Clin Pharmacol 1989;29:272–7.

[10] Marik PE. The treatment of hypoalbuminemia in the critically ill patient. Heart Lung 1993;22:166–70.

[11] Vree TB, Shimoda M, Driessen JJ, et al. Decreased plasma albumin concentration results in increased volume of distribution and decreased elimination of midazolam in intensive care patients. Clin Pharmacol Ther 1989;46:537–44.

[12] Haberer JP, Schoeffler P, Couderc E, et al. Fentanyl pharmacokinetics in anaesthetized patients with cirrhosis. Br J Anaesth 1982;54:1267–70.

[13] Child CG. The liver and portal hypertension. Philadelphia: WB Saunders; 1964.

[14] Pugh RN, Murray-Lyon IM, Dawson JL, et al. Transection of the oesophagus for bleeding oesophageal varices. Br J Surg 1973;60:646–9.

[15] Kamath PS, Wiesner RH, Malinchoc M, et al. A model to predict survival in patients with end-stage liver disease. Hepatology 2001;33:464–70.

[16] Davies G, Kingswood C, Street M. Pharmacokinetics of opioids in renal dysfunction. Clin Pharmacokinet 1996;31:410–22.

[17] Klotz U. Pathophysiological and disease-induced changes in drug distribution volume: pharmacokinetic implications. Clin Pharmacokinet 1976;1:204–18.

[18] Vree TB, Hekster YA, Anderson PG. Contribution of the human kidney to the metabolic clearance of drugs. Ann Pharmacother 1992;26:1421–8.

[19] Gibson TP. Renal disease and drug metabolism: an overview. Am J Kidney Dis 1986;8:7–17.

[20] Anders MW. Metabolism of drugs by the kidney. Kidney Int 1980;18:636–47.

[21] Milne RW, Nation RL, Somogyi AA, et al. The influence of renal function on the renal clearance of morphine and its glucuronide metabolites in intensive-care patients. Br J Clin Pharmacol 1992; 34:53–9.

[22] Bauer TM, Ritz R, Haberthur C, et al. Prolonged sedation due to accumulation of conjugated metabolites of midazolam. Lancet 1995;346:145–7.

[23] Morrison G, Chiang ST, Koepke HH, et al. Effect of renal impairment and hemodialysis on lorazepam kinetics. Clin Pharmacol Ther 1984;35:646–52.

[24] Jelliffe RW. Estimation of creatinine clearance when urine cannot be collected. Lancet 1971;1:975–6.

[25] Jelliffe RW. Letter: creatinine clearance: bedside estimate. Ann Intern Med 1973;79:604–5.

[26] Levey AS, Bosch JP, Lewis JB, et al. A more accurate method to estimate glomerular filtration rate from serum creatinine: a new prediction equation. Modification of Diet in Renal Disease Study Group. Ann Intern Med 1999;130:461–70.

[27] Gaspari F, Ferrari S, Stucchi N, et al. Performance of different prediction equations for estimating renal function in kidney transplantation. Am J Transplant 2004;4:1826–35.

[28] Cockcroft DW, Gault MH. Prediction of creatinine clearance from serum creatinine. Nephron 1976;16: 31–41.

[29] Sherman DS, Fish DN, Teitelbaum I. Assessing renal function in cirrhotic patients: problems and pitfalls. Am J Kidney Dis 2003;41:269–78.

[30] Jacobi J, Fraser GL, Coursin DB, et al. Clinical practice guidelines for the sustained use of sedatives and analgesics in the critically ill adult. Crit Care Med 2002;30:119–41.

[31] Watson BD, Kane-Gill SL. Sedation assessment in critically ill adults: 2001–2004 update. Ann Pharmacother 2004;38:1898–906.

[32] Deogaonkar A, Gupta R, Degeorgia M, et al. Bispectral Index monitoring correlates with sedation scales in brain-injured patients. Crit Care Med 2004; 32:2403–6.

ELSEVIER
SAUNDERS

CRITICAL CARE
NURSING CLINICS
OF NORTH AMERICA

Crit Care Nurs Clin N Am 17 (2005) 251 – 255

Sleep in Mechanically Ventilated Patients

Judith L. Reishtein, PhD, RN

*School of Nursing and Center for Sleep and Respiratory Neurobiology, University of Pennsylvania, Nursing Education Building,
420 Guardian Drive, Philadelphia, PA 19104, USA*

Hospitals are infamous as places where people cannot sleep, and critical care units seem to be the worst offenders in denying their guests rest and sleep. Patients who leave the critical care environment are so sleep deprived, they often spend the next 2 or 3 days sleeping for prolonged periods, alarming their families and naive nursing staff. Aside from this sleep deprivation, however, very little is known about sleep in critically ill patients, especially in those who are dependent on mechanical ventilation [1,2].

Normal sleep

Normal sleep, as experienced by healthy people, can be divided into several stages, based on electroencephalogram (EEG) waves. Stage 1 is not actually sleep, but the period of drowsiness during which the brain waves slow, just as a person is falling asleep; it is a relatively short period (about 2%–5% of total sleep time), and the person can wake from it easily (Table 1). Most sleep time is spent in stage 2, light sleep, which is characterized on an EEG by "sleep spindles." During stage 2 sleep, the individual is unresponsive to stimuli. Stages 3 and 4, called slow wave sleep because of the appearance of the associated EEG waves, are deep sleep. During slow

wave sleep, although muscle tone is present, there is no movement, and both breathing and the heart rate are slow and steady. Rapid eye movement (REM) sleep, named for its characteristic eye movements, is identified by rapid waves on the EEG, muscle atonia, and increased and variable heart and respiratory rates. REM sleep is associated with dreaming. Sleep progresses in a predictable fashion through the stages, taking about 90 minutes for each cycle through the four stages and REM.

The regularity of sleep is a manifestation of circadian rhythm, the approximately 24-hour cycling of the body clock. This clock is synchronized daily by exposure to light and by regular occurrences, such as meals and social activity. When the circadian clock is malfunctioning, because of illness, jet lag, shift work, or constant exposure to light, the individual has difficulty sleeping. Because many hormones (eg, cortisol, thyroid-stimulating hormone, melatonin) are secreted according to daily rhythms, disruption of circadian rhythm and sleep can lead to problems in almost all body systems.

Sleep is necessary for proper physiologic function. Most growth hormone, necessary for proper healing, is secreted during sleep, and cortisol secretion increases just before awakening. Slow wave sleep is associated with increases in immunologic activity. Cognitive function also depends on sleep. Sleep deprivation can cause memory lapses, increased reaction time, decreased alertness, and reduced learning ability. People who are critically ill are especially vulnerable to some of the effects of sleep deprivation, especially poorer immune function, increases in both carbon dioxide production and oxygen use, and negative nitrogen balance [3–5].

This work was supported by grant number 5-T32-HL07953-03 from the National Institutes of Health.
E-mail address: reishtei@nursing.upenn.edu

Table 1
Characteristics of sleep in mechanically ventilated and non-mechanically ventilated people

	Freedman et al [1] (2001) 24 hours N = 17	Gabor et al [13] (2001) 24 hours N = 7	Cooper et al [12] (2000) Disrupted sleep mean (SD) N = 8		Cooper et al [12] (2000) Atypical sleep mean (SD) N = 5		Carskadon and Dement [20] (2000) Normal mean
			Day	Night	Day	Night	
Total sleep hours	8.8 (5)	6.2 (2.5)	4 (2.9)	3 (1.9)	6 (3)	4 (2)	—
Stage 1%	59 (33)	19 (6.6)	43 (26)	40 (28)	36 (36)	37 (42)	2–5
Stage 2%	26 (28)*	64 (10)	33 (18)	40 (23)	*	*	45–55
Stage 3 and 4 (SWS)%	9 (18)	2.7 (3.3)	15 (14)	10 (17)	46 (47)	45 (51)	13–23
REM%	6 (9)*	14.3 (9.8)	9 (6)	10 (14)	*	*	20–25
Arousals plus wakenings per hour	—	21.7 (7.6)	42	42	14	12	—

Abbreviations: REM, rapid eye movement; SD, standard deviation; SWS, slow wave sleep.
  * These stages did not occur in all patients.

Changes in these functions can prolong their illness, lead to additional complications, and delay weaning from mechanical ventilation.

Problems related to research on mechanically ventilated patients

Few studies of sleep have been conducted in mechanically ventilated patients because of ethical and methodologic issues. Patients in critical care units, because they are physically restricted and dependent on hospital staff, are considered captive and vulnerable, and in need of special protection.

Each participant in health research must be informed about the purpose of the study, the procedures to be performed, and its possible benefits and harmful effects. Most patients receiving mechanical ventilatory support cannot give consent because either their disease process or their medications interfere with their ability to evaluate information and make decisions [6]. It is difficult to assess a mechanically ventilated person's ability to understand and consent to a research protocol; only one study has documented the process of obtaining consent in ventilated patients [7]. If the participant cannot give consent, consent must be obtained from the person making decisions for him or her, usually a family member. Many family members are so overwhelmed by the experience of seeing a loved one in the critical care unit, they have difficulty giving consent for necessary procedures, let alone one that provides no immediate benefit. Alternatively, some family members may feel pressured to give consent because they be-

lieve doing so will ensure their loved one of receiving good care [6].

Assuming consent can be obtained, actually performing a sleep study, or polysomnogram (PSG), in a critical care room is fraught with problems. In addition to ECG and oximetry, which are already being monitored in the critically ill patient, a PSG requires four EEG leads on the head to detect brain waves, and recording equipment. If the patient is not paralyzed by drugs, the PSG also includes electromyogram leads under the chin to detect muscle tension, electro-oculogram leads at the corner of each eye to detect eye movement, and sensors for detecting body position and leg movement. The standard PSG also records air flow at the nose and chest and abdominal respiratory movements, which are meaningless in a mechanically ventilated patient. Even the most basic recording equipment and fewest leads take up space and complicate patient care. Additonally, space must be made for the monitoring equipment and the PSG technologist.

Subjective evaluations of sleep

Subjective assessments of sleep following extubation and discharge from critical care is difficult because patients have poor time sense and recall of what happened [8]. In one group of 20 patients who had been dependant on mechanical ventilation for 7 days or more, several indicated they had difficulty remembering what their sleep and rest had been like. When they rated their sleep on the Verran Snyder-Halpern Sleep Scale, many values were missing, and two of the three subscales had only poor to fair reliability [8]. When patients' ratings of their sleep on the Verran Snyder-Halpern Sleep Scale were compared with PSG measurements, the Verran Snyder-Halpern Sleep Scale scores had small nonsignificant correlations with the PSG measurements of time to fall asleep (sleep latency) and time spent awake after sleep onset [9]. When subjective evaluations of sleep were compared, ventilator patients complained of more daytime sleepiness than nonventilator patients [10].

Some patients receive heavy sedation or are paralyzed while on the ventilator either to prevent ventilator dysynchrony or to ensure patient rest and relief from anxiety. This therapy can disrupt both sleep and memory of the intensive care episode. Occasionally, however, a recovered patient can give the health care team insight into the ventilator experience. One patient stated that while she was on the ventilator, paralyzed and sedated, she had very vivid dreams and because of what the people in her dreams were saying, she had thought she was dead. When informed by the nurses that they had told her, several times every day, that she was alive and was being cared for, she replied, "But I didn't hear it from the people in my dreams. They were the only ones I could hear" (personal communication, 1998).

Another type of subjective evaluation is the health care worker's assessment of a patient's sleep. When nurses' assessments were compared with simultaneous PSG recordings of six patients in intensive care, the nurses consistently overestimated the amount of sleep the patients were experiencing, often by large amounts [11]. Nurses' assessments of sleep latency and time spent awake after sleep onset were moderately related to PSG measurements of these times ($r = .37$ and 0.59, respectively, both $P < .05$) [9].

Objective evaluations of sleep

Four groups of researchers used PSG to monitor mechanically ventilated patients for 24 or more hours. Not one patient experienced normal sleep (see Table 1). Although some patients experienced the traditionally "normal" 8 hours of sleep over the course of 24 hours, half of the sleep time occurred during the daytime. All the patients had more light (stage 1) sleep and less REM sleep than normal.

A sample of 20 mechanically ventilated patients consisted of three groups: (1) those with disrupted sleep, (2) those with atypical sleep, and (3) those in a coma. The eight patients with disrupted sleep were significantly less sick than the other patients. They had better scores on the Apache II Physiologic Scale (6 ± 4 versus 13 ± 4), the Glasgow Coma Score (14 ± 3 versus 8 ± 3), and the Lung Injury Scale (1.8 ± 0.6 versus 1.7 ± 1.1), and had spent significantly less time in the ICU (9 ± 11 versus 10 ± 6 days; all $P < .05$). Disrupted sleep differed from normal sleep in several ways. There was more stage 1 (light) sleep and less REM (dreaming) sleep than in age-matched controls (as reported in other studies), but similar to what has been reported in other acutely ill populations. Sleep was very fragmented, with patients arousing or waking 17 to 22 times an hour. In contrast, the five atypical sleepers slept more over the course of 24 hours, but experienced virtually no stage 2 or REM sleep, going directly from light sleep to deep slow wave sleep. They also experienced pathologic wakefulness, in which behaviors that are normally found only during wakefulness, such as muscle tension, occurred when the EEG indicated they were in deep slow wave sleep. When the atypical group did sleep, they also roused or woke frequently (14–15 times an hour) [12].

The sleep of seven mechanically ventilated men averaged 6.2 (± 2.5) hours, only half of which occurred at night. This was compared with normal volunteers who spent a day in the same critical care unit, who averaged 8.2 (± 1.4) hours, 70% during the night (see Table 1). Because the study did not have enough subjects (power = .35), however, the results were not significant [13].

A study of 17 mechanically ventilated, non-sedated, noncomatose ICU patients who were continuously monitored by PSG for 24 or 48 hours found similar sleep patterns. The patients slept at all hours around the clock, with 57% (± 18) of sleep during normal waking hours (6 AM–10 PM). Sleep frequently occurred in short bursts (15 $\pm$ 9 minutes); was frequently disrupted (11.6 arousals per hour); and its architecture was abnormal (see Table 1) [1].

Causes of impaired sleep

Frequent disruptions of sleep not only decrease total sleep time, but also interfere with normal progression and distribution of sleep stages. For sleep to be effective, appropriate time must be spent in each stage. For example, without sufficient slow wave sleep and REM, memories cannot be moved into long-term storage for later retrieval.

Postulated causes of disrupted sleep in the critical care unit include ventilator dysynchrony, noise, interventions related to care, pain, anxiety, underlying acute or chronic disease, circadian rhythm disturbances, light, noxious odors, and effects of medications [1,12,14].

Because of all the equipment, alarms, and staff conversations, ICUs are fairly noisy places, even at night. Ambient noise in ICU has measured at between 60 and 84 dB over 24 hours. In one hospital, sound levels were greater than 80 dB between 150 and 200 times during the night [15]. In comparison, an alarm clock is about 65 to 80 dB, vacuum cleaners and power mowers average 60 to 85 dB, and freeway traffic is about 70 dB [16]. The Environmental Protection Agency recommends hospital sound levels should not be above 45 dB during the day and 35 dB at night (similar to a quiet office). When ambient noise was measured during 24-hour PSG, it was discovered that noise was responsible for only 11.5% of all arousals and 17% of all awakenings, or a mean of 26% of awakenings per subject [1]. More arousals and awakenings are caused by patient care interactions. Tamburri and colleagues [17] found a mean of 42.6 care interactions with each patient per night. Over the course of 147 patient nights, they found only nine instances of a patient being uninterrupted for 2 hours, and not one instance of three interruption-free hours. Because a sleep cycle is 1.5 to 2 hours, normal sleep architecture is disrupted by patient care.

Why do critically ill patients experience no REM sleep? Several reasons have been proposed: bursts of sleep are too short to allow progression into REM; circadian rhythm, which controls timing of REM periods, is disturbed; presence of inflammatory mediators, which inhibit REM sleep; or use of REM inhibiting drugs [1]. Freedman and colleagues [1] argue against drug action being the exclusive reason because most of their patients did not take any REM-suppressing medication.

Even when efforts are made to decrease sleep-disrupting external stimuli and to keep patients as pain free as possible, they do not sleep well. One researcher limited noise, light, and nursing activities as much as possible (especially at night), and he remained in the unit almost constantly. Nevertheless, the nine patients being monitored slept an average of only 139 minutes on their second day in the ICU [11]. This seems to indicate that there is something intrinsic about critical illness that interferes with sleep.

Sepsis may interfere with sleep, independently of any other sleep-disrupting factor. Although Cooper and colleagues [12] stated that none of the people in their study had bacteremia, those with atypical sleep exhibited a pattern similar to that of septic patients in another study [12]. Mechanically ventilated patients who became septic had no definable markers of either stage 2 or REM sleep on their EEGs. These changes in sleep were detectable on the PSG up to 8 hours before any signs of sepsis became apparent [1].

Recommendations

The paucity of research on sleep in patients who require mechanical ventilation is a problem for health care workers. Without more definitive information, it is difficult, if not impossible, to develop guidelines for optimal care of these people. Some of the few studies that have been performed [11,18,19] warrant replication because they are over 10 years old. Methods of studying sleep have advanced and ventilator technology has changed in ways that may invalidate the conclusions of earlier studies. More research is needed to pinpoint the exact causes of poor sleep in this vulnerable group.

Even without further information, however, caregivers can use current knowledge as the basis for action. Caregiving activities have been demonstrated to be major sleep disrupting factors in the ICU. It is important for nurses and others to avoid performing such activities when the patient might be sleeping. Because it has been demonstrated that nurses are not good judges of when a patient is actually asleep, it is appropriate to avoid unnecessary activities for the duration of the usual hours of sleep. Decreasing noise and light during the nighttime hours is also helpful in maintaining the patients' normal circadian rhythms and promoting sleep. Because at least half of patients' sleep occurs during the daylight hours, it is advisable to keep noise levels low during the daytime, and to group patient care activities to allow uninterrupted time for sleep during the daytime.

Summary

People who are undergoing mechanical ventilation in an ICU sleep poorly. Only half of their sleep occurs in what are normal sleep hours (10:00 PM – 6:00 AM). The architecture is aberrant, with occasional disappearance of stage 2 or REM sleep altogether, and there are frequent arousals and awakenings. Because the largest proportion of arousals are associated with caregiving activities and noise, it would improve patient sleep patterns if caregivers consolidate care so as not to disturb patients, and to eliminate or dampen as many sources of noise as possible. More research is needed on sleep and its promotion in mechanically ventilated patients.

References

[1] Freedman NS, Gazendam J, Levan L, et al. Abnormal sleep/wake cycles and the effect of environmental noise on sleep disruption in the intensive care unit. Am J Respir Crit Care Med 2001;163:451–7.

[2] Krachman SL, D'Alonzo GE, Criner GJ. Sleep in the intensive care unit. Chest 1995;107:1713–20.

[3] Benca RM, Quintas J. Sleep and host defenses: a review. Sleep 1997;20:1027–37.

[4] Bonnet MH, Berry RB, Arand DL. Metabolism during normal, fragmented, and recovery sleep. J Appl Physiol 1991;71:1112–8.

[5] Scrimshaw NS, Habicht JP, Pellet P, et al. Effects of sleep deprivation and reversal of diurnal activity on protein metabolism of young men. Am J Clin Nutr 1966;19:313–9.

[6] Society AT. The ethical conduct of clinical research involving critically ill patients in the United States and Canada: principles and recommendations. Am J Respir Crit Care Med 2004;170:1375–84.

[7] Higgins PA, Daly BJ. Research methodology issues related to interviewing the mechanically ventilated patient. West J Nurs Res 1999;21:773–84.

[8] Higgins PA. Patient perception of fatigue while undergoing long-term mechanical ventilation: incidence and associated factors. Heart Lung 1998;27:177–83.

[9] Fontaine DK. Measurement of nocturnal sleep patterns in trauma patients. Heart Lung 1989;18:402–10.

[10] Freedman NS, Kotzer N, Schwab RJ. Patient perception of sleep quality and etiology of sleep disruption in the intensive care unit. Am J Respir Crit Care Med 1999;159:1155–62.

[11] Aurell J, Elmqvist D. Sleep in the surgical intensive care unit: continuous polygraphic recording of sleep in nine patients receiving postoperative care. BMJ 1985; 290:1029–32.

[12] Cooper AB, Thornley KS, Young GB, et al. Sleep in critically ill patients requiring mechanical ventilation. Chest 2000;117:809–18.

[13] Gabor JY, Cooper AB, Crombach SA, et al. Contribution of the intensive care unit environment to sleep disruption in mechanically ventilated patients and healthy subjects. Am J Respir Crit Care Med 2003; 167:708–15.

[14] Gabor JY, Cooper AB, Hanly PJ. Sleep disruption in the intensive care unit. Curr Opin Crit Care 2001;7: 21–7.

[15] Aaron JN, Carlisle CC, Carskadon MA, et al. Environmental noise as a cause of sleep disruption in an intermediate respiratory care unit. Sleep 1996;19:707–10.

[16] League for the Hard of Hearing. Noise center of the league: noise levels in our environment. Available at: www/lhh.org/noise/decibel.htm. Accessed December 20, 2004.

[17] Tamburri LM, DiBrienza R, Zozula R, et al. Nocturnal care interactions with patients in critical care units. Am J Crit Care 2004;13:102–12.

[18] Broughton R, Baron R. Sleep patterns in the intensive care unit and on the ward after acute myocardial infarction. Electroencephalogr Clin Neurophysiol 1978;45:348–60.

[19] Helton MC, Gordon SH, Nunnery SL. The correlation between sleep deprivation and the intensive care unit syndrome. Heart Lung 1980;9:464–8.

[20] Carskadon MA, Dement WC. Normal human sleep: an overview. In: Kryger M, Roth T, Dement WC, editors. Principles and practice of sleep medicine. Philadelphia: WB Saunders; 2000. p. 15–25.

ELSEVIER
SAUNDERS

Crit Care Nurs Clin N Am 17 (2005) 257 – 267

CRITICAL CARE
NURSING CLINICS
OF NORTH AMERICA

Toward Solving the Sedation-Assessment Conundrum: Bispectral Index Monitoring and Sedation Interruption

DaiWai M. Olson, RN, BSN, CCRN[a,b,*], Carmelo Graffagnino, MD[b], Kenneth King, RN, BSN[c], John R. Lynch, MD[b]

[a]The University of North Carolina at Chapel Hill, School of Nursing, Carrington Hall, Campus Box 7460, Chapel Hill, NC 27599-7460, USA
[b]Department of Internal Medicine, Duke University Medical Center, Erwin Road, Durham, NC 27710, USA
[c]Duke University Medical Center, Erwin Road, Durham, NC 27710, USA

Two vital but opposing forces exist in the intensive care setting: the need to maintain a state of adequate sedation balanced against the need to obtain a comprehensive neurologic examination. This presents practitioners with two diametrically opposed goals that lead to the sedation-assessment conundrum: to maintain a level of sedation that facilitates ventilatory and hemodynamic stability within a safe environment, and to ensure that the neurologic examination obtained represents the patient's best effort and most accurate reflection of the patient's neurologic status [1–3]. It is imperative to know whether any deficits appreciated in the neurologic examination are related to the patient's altered neurologic function rather than caused by the chemically depressed level of consciousness [4]. Supplementing subjective sedation assessment with bispectral (BIS) index monitoring facilitates a more comprehensive understanding of the patient's sedation status.

Case presentation

A 61-year-old man with a past medical history of coronary artery disease, hypertension, and peripheral vascular disease presents with acute worsening of vascular claudication secondary to a thrombosed lower extremity arterial bypass graft. In an effort to salvage the ischemic leg he received intra-arterial thrombolytic therapy with tissue plasminogen activator. At the conclusion of the intervention he was admitted to the surgical ICU for follow-up observation and treatment. A stat CT scan of his brain was obtained when he failed to wake up from his general anesthetic. The CT scan revealed a large right occipital-parietal intraparenchymal hemorrhage. This was surgically evacuated by an open craniotomy and he was admitted directly to the neuroscience critical care unit following surgery.

At the time of arrival to the neuroscience critical care unit he was orally intubated and required ventilatory support. The anesthetist reported that the patient had been sedated with remifentanil and propofol before leaving the operating room. In the neuroscience critical care unit the patient was immediately placed on full mechanical ventilatory support, bedside cardiac monitor, and intra-arterial blood pressure monitoring. The nurse and resident physician completed the initial physical assessment and continued to monitor the patient's hemodynamic status.

As the effects of sedation began to wear off, the patient became dangerously agitated. He attempted to climb out of bed and remove his endotracheal tube while kicking his legs violently. This increased state of arousal was associated with an increased blood pressure (178/56 mm Hg) and heart rate (128 beats

This research is supported by T32 NR07091 Interventions to Prevent and Manage Chronic Illness.

* Corresponding author. 3 Gamble Court, Durham, NC 27712.

E-mail address: dmOlson@email.unc.edu (D.M. Olson).

per minute). Mechanical ventilation became difficult as a result of the violent head shaking, asynchronous breathing, and biting down on the endotracheal tube. This patient was clearly at increased risk of complications from uncontrolled hypertension, tachycardia, and increased intracranial pressure. Extubation was not an option because the patient did not meet criteria for spontaneous breathing.

At this time, it was determined that the patient required analgesia and sedation to facilitate continued mechanical ventilation. Propofol was chosen as the sedative agent because of its favorable pharmacokinetic properties (rapid onset of action, short half-life, and predictable dose-response curve). Depth of sedation was objectively monitored using a BIS monitor (Model A2000XP, Aspect Medical Systems, Natick, Massachusetts), with the goal of maintaining a BIS score between 60 and 70 [5]. He was subjectively monitored with a modified version of the Ramsay Scale; the sedation goal was to maintain a modified Ramsay score of 3 or 4. Shortly after the propofol infusion was initiated, the patient's agitation subsided, manifested by a decrease in heart rate, blood pressure, and respiratory rate. It is important to note that at this level of sedation a reliable and reproducible neurologic examination was still possible. When it became necessary to assess a more comprehensive level of neurologic function, the propofol was slowly weaned down to a rate that produced a BIS score between 80 and 85. This level of sedation allowed the patient to be able to follow more complex commands and cooperate with a detailed neurologic examination. The ability clinically to monitor this patient on such a close basis allowed the nurse to discover that the patient had developed a number of new focal neurologic deficits including a left mouth droop, a diminished left corneal reflex, a weakened left gag reflex, and a left upper extremity drift. All of these findings had not been appreciated during the earlier examination when the patient had been in a highly agitated state or heavier level of sedation. Eventually, the patient improved from his acute neurologic injury and the depth of sedation was likewise decreased, allowing the patient to be safely extubated.

Defining the sedation-assessment conundrum

This case presentation illustrates the sedation-assessment conundrum. This patient required sedation to meet his medical management goals; controlling the ill effects of agitation, elevated blood pressure, and increased heart rate and maintaining adequate mechanical ventilation. Yet, to obtain a comprehensive neurologic assessment to identify any new deficits, the sedatives needed to be discontinued. Although sedatives could not be stopped, it was possible to titrate sedation tightly to minimize the hemodynamic and intracranial instability that happens at lower levels of sedation. Sedation does not have to be an all or none phenomenon; rather, it is a continuum. This was accomplished using a combination of sound subjective assessment skills combined with the objectivity of the BIS monitor.

Sedation goals

Sedation, paralysis, and analgesia remain separate, yet often intertwined concerns [6]. When discussing sedation it is important to recognize that the sedation goal is a two-tiered goal. The primary goal is the "why" goal, or the reason for sedation. The secondary goal is the "how much" goal. The individualized patient need for sedation, the "why," drives the decision to determine the desired degree of sedation, the "how much." In 2002, the American Society of Health Systems Pharmacists and American College of Critical Care Medicine, Society of Critical Care Medicine, developed a set of guidelines for sedation assessment and monitoring [7]. A key aspect among these guidelines is the need to set and regularly redefine the goal of sedation. In the intensive care setting, there are a variety of reasons why one might sedate a patient. Three of the primary indications for sedation are (1) injury prevention, (2) facilitation of medical goals, and (3) humanitarian goals [8,9].

The first reason is that the patient, if left without adequate sedation, may cause injury to themselves or others. This may include removal of medically necessary monitoring or support devices and causing injury to the staff members caring for them while in a state of delirium. A second reason for sedating a patient is to facilitate the medical goals set for the patient. This includes maintaining hemodynamic stability, increasing ventilatory compliance, and controlling intracranial pressure [10]. The third reason for sedating a patient is for humanitarian intentions. All patients treated with neuromuscular blocking agents should be concurrently sedated to avoid the emotional distress associated with total body paralysis [11]. Adequate sedation of the critically ill patient also becomes paramount when an individual is inflicted with a barrage of noxious stimuli and invasive procedures, such as the insertion of intracranial pressure monitoring devices or placement of medically necessary catheters and monitoring devices. Adequate sedation, depending on the agent, results in a degree of induced amnesia for the events associated with the intensive care experience, protecting the patient against the long-term emotional stress of the acute illness [12]. Although each of these three reasons individually provides justification for sedation, often the needs overlap.

Once the decision is made to use sedation, the depth and goals of sedation must then be determined, which should be clearly communicated among those prescribing and those titrating the sedating agent [6]. The use of a subjective in conjunction with an objective assessment tool is indicated to monitor the level of sedation [13–15]. The depth of sedation is, in part, determined by the sedation scales or tools used [6,16]. A variety of subjective sedation assessment tools have been developed and tested with varying degrees of validity and reliability that use some form of numerical reference [17–23].

The sedation goal must be individualized to the patient's need for sedation [9]. If the indication for sedation is one of injury prevention a lighter state of sedation is likely indicated, such that the patient is cooperative but is able to communicate with the staff [6]. If the indication for sedation is to facilitate an individual medical goal, the sedation level may need to be somewhat deeper [9]. The most challenging situation involving sedation is the one in which the indication for sedation is for humanitarian needs. There is wide variability in providing adequate depth of sedation for the purpose of comfort. Sedation for palliative care may range from mild to deep sedation based on the individual desires of the patient and family [6,24,25]. For a patient who is chemically paralyzed it is highly undesirable to experience an awakened state; a deeper level of sedation is indicated.

Sedation challenges

Achieving and maintaining a specific sedation goal requires nursing vigilance. Patient response to medication is often unpredictable and varies not only within and between patient populations, but also within a single hospital stay for an individual patient. Drug accumulation; changes in hemodynamic status; changes in renal, endocrine, and liver function; and the effects of drug-to-drug interaction can increase or decrease the effectiveness of sedating agents [9]. The challenge of maintaining appropriate goals without

oversedation or undersedation, while allowing the monitoring of a patient's neurologic examination, requires the nurse to be skillful in incorporating subjective and objective data.

Oversedation

Oversedation is common to many intensive care settings and may result from poorly used or poorly validated scales [26]. Oversedation may also occur as a result of different methods of intravenous administration, continuous or bolus. Long-term sedation in the critical care setting is most often achieved by the use of a continuous infusion of a sedative agent, often with concurrent administration of analgesic agents that may have synergistic drug effects often resulting in a decreased level of consciousness. It is critical that the nurse be certain whether an individual patient requires increased analgesia to reduce pain or whether it is sedation that is required, prompting an increase in the sedative drug. Too often analgesics are used interchangeably as sedatives, failing to meet the patient's need for a balance of pain control and sedation. Increased length of mechanical ventilation, decreased wound healing, and decreased gastrointestinal motility have all been attributed to oversedation in the critical care setting [27–29]. Recently, the use of high-dose propofol has been linked with an increased incidence of rhabdomyolysis, cardiac failure, metabolic acidosis, and renal failure, although these complications are more common in children than adults [30–32]. Oversedation may impair the reliability of the neurologic examination particularly when the evaluating individual is less experienced [3,4]. In contrast to the use of continuous infusions, patients managed with bolus dosing have been shown to have significantly higher scores on the Sedation-Agitation Scale (more agitated) and higher BIS scores (more alert) than patients receiving continuous infusions of sedatives and hypnotics [33]. This results in higher doses of both sedative and analgesic drugs being used to achieve the same sedation goals.

Undersedation

Although undersedation is less common to the critical care setting than oversedation, the morbidity associated with undersedation can be quite profound [26]. Inadequate sedation can lead to decreased patient safety and increased risk of injury. Compromised patient safety as a result of undersedation is most easily manifest in the example of patients removing intravenous or intra-arterial lines, and unplanned self-extubation [34,35]. Boulain [34], in a prospective observational study, evaluated the incidence of unplanned self-extubation and found that inadequate sedation was one of four associated factors. Undersedation may contribute to ventilatory asynchrony, patient movement during procedures, and episodes of hemodynamic and intracranial instability [5]. Few studies have examined the incidence of recall of unpleasant events within the critical care setting. Cheng [36], however, suggests that improved sedation and sedation monitoring decrease the incidence of unpleasant recall in the ICU setting [37].

Some of the difficulty in optimizing sedation may be attributed to the complexity of drug selection and drug combinations available. Criteria for drug selection are not well defined [38,39]. A wide variety of medications exist that can be used as sedating agents either singly, or in conjunction with other medications [7,40]. Central-acting sedatives alter the effects of key neurotransmitters. In the central nervous system (CNS) the major neurotransmitters involved in regulating consciousness are γ-aminobutyric acid (GABA) and glutamate [1,41]. GABA is an inhibitory neurotransmitter; glutamate is an excitatory neurotransmitter [42]. Benzodiazepines are one of the most common classes of medication used for sedation. Two of the primary benzodiazepines used in the ICU setting are midazolam and lorazepam. Midazolam interacts with receptors in the CNS to increase the inhibitory effect of GABA, which produces an anxiolytic, sedative effect [43]. Lorazepam, like midazolam, globally depresses the CNS function by increasing the effects of GABA but has a longer half-life [44]. Benzodiazepines, such as lorazepam, are metabolized in the liver by being rapidly conjugated at the 3-hydroxy group into lorazepam glucuronide (inactive in the CNS), which is then excreted by the kidneys [45].

Propofol is a phospholipid-based parentally administered anesthetic that is metabolized in the liver and excreted by the kidneys [46,47]. Propofol inhibits the N-methyl-D-aspartate subtype of glutamate receptors by channel gating modulation and has agonistic activity at the GABA receptors [45].

Propofol has a relatively short half-life with sedative effects generally lasting from 4 to 8 minutes when used in doses of 1.5 to 2.5 mg/kg/h, although the pharmacokinetic effect of propofol has been shown to be dependent in part on body weight and fat content [47–49]. Despite propofol having a higher cost per dosage than short-acting benzodiazepines, such as midazolam [38], its use as a sedative in mechanically ventilated patients has actually been shown to decrease the overall cost of care because of the relatively short half-life of the drug, which facilitates a shorter time to extubation [38,50]. The use of high-dose propofol for prolonged periods should be avoided, however, because of the increased risk for the development of pancreatitis, cardiac failure, metabolic acidosis, renal failure, and rhabdomyolysis [30].

Barbiturates, such as pentobarbital and phenobarbital, and opiates, such as morphine and fentanyl, are often used in conjunction with primary acting sedatives. Barbiturates, which act as nonselective depressants of the CNS, are capable of producing all levels of CNS mood alteration, ranging from excitation to mild sedation, hypnosis, and deep coma [45]. The sedative-hypnotic and anticonvulsant properties of barbiturates may be related to their ability to enhance or mimic the inhibitory synaptic action of GABA, interfering with the transmission of excitatory impulses from the thalamus to the cerebral cortex. Although metabolized in the liver and excreted by the kidneys, phenobarbital has a relatively long and unpredictable half-life ranging from 30 to 140 hours in adults [51,52]. Phenobarbital and pentobarbital are nearly homonyms, a fact that can lead to significant confusion. Because pentobarbital has a half-life of 35 to 50 hours in adults, it is considered a shorter-acting barbiturate than its counterpart phenobarbital. Pentobarbital is almost completely metabolized in the liver [53].

Opiates, such as heroin and morphine, are derived from the sap of the poppy seed pod. Newer agents, such as hydromorphone, fentanyl, remifentanil, hydrocodone, and codeine, have been pharmacologically synthesized. All of these agents bind to opiate receptors (Mu receptors) in the CNS, which results in an inhibition of ascending pain pathways and altering pain perception and response to pain. All of the opiates are metabolized in the liver and variably excreted by the kidneys [54].

Hydromorphone is one of the most potent opiate analgesics available and has a half-life of 1 to 3 hours [45]. Heroin is rarely used pharmacologically as an analgesic agent in the United States; however, it is legally used in the United Kingdom and a few other countries to control symptoms of cancer. Heroin has a rapid onset of intense euphoria from high lipid solubility provided by the two acetyl groups, resulting in a very rapid penetration of the blood-brain barrier after parenteral administration; in the brain, heroin is rapidly metabolized into morphine by oxidation of the acetyl groups [55]. Morphine, however, is the most commonly used parenteral analgesic agent. Its duration of action is 1 to 3 hours [56].

Fentanyl, a newer short-acting opiate, has a half-life of 2 to 4 hours [57]. Remifentanil is extremely short-acting and cleared by nonspecific esterases located primarily in muscle and intestines. It has a half-life of 6 minutes and an elimination half-life of 10 to 20 minutes and is most often used during surgical interventions [45]. The two most commonly used oral analgesics are codeine and hydrocodone. Both of these agents can be used alone or in combination with acetaminophen or aspirin. Codeine is metabolized to morphine. Its duration of action is 4 to 6 hours [58]. Opiates are primarily used as analgesics, but when used in sufficiently high doses they may produce a sedation-like side effect [59].

Dexmedetomidine is a relatively new drug being used for sedation in the critical care setting. Dexmedetomidine is a α_2-adrenoreceptor agonist with a combination of sedative and analgesic effects [60]. Activation of the α_2-adrenoreceptor sites within the CNS produces an inhibition in the stress response, thereby facilitating sedation. Dexmedetomidine is administered as a continuous intravenous infusion not to exceed 24 hours. The elimination half-life is stated as 2 hours [61].

Although understanding the mechanism of action for various sedatives and analgesics is vitally important, this knowledge only allows for ensuring that each medication is prescribed and delivered at a correct dosage level. The most important decision when choosing a sedative or analgesic agent is to understand the specific indication for use at the time the medication is prescribed. The practitioner must be cognizant of why each medication is being used, along with the needs of the patient at the time. If the reason for sedation is one of facilitating humanitarian goals it may be that a longer-acting sedative is indicated. If the patient is acutely critically ill and requires close hemodynamic and physiologic monitoring, then it is likely that the sedation needs frequent adjustment. In the case of obtaining a neurologic examination, interruption to allow the patient to awaken from the effects of sedation is needed, in which case a shorter-acting agent is ideal.

The neurologic examination

The purpose of the neurologic examination is to evaluate the functional status of the nervous system. This examination begins with an assessment of the higher cortical functions, such as level of consciousness and cognition. Level of consciousness is judged according to the amount of stimulus required to have the patient perform actions, such as eye opening and engaging the examiner. Once a patient is considered to be conscious (responsive and reactive to stimuli), specific cortical functions are tested, such as language (spoken and receptive), orientation, cooperation. Higher motor and sensory functions are then tested. The combination of the ability to open eyes, speak, and follow motor commands constitutes the sub-components of the Glasgow Coma Score [62]. This scale was designed for use in monitoring the neuro-cognitive status of a patient with traumatic brain injury. When used for other conditions, such as spinal cord injury, sedation assessment, or vascular neurologic injury (hemorrhagic and ischemic stroke), the Glasgow Coma Score loses its specificity and sensitivity as a monitoring tool. When a patient is noted to have an impaired level of consciousness it is critical to determine whether this has resulted from a focal lesion impairing the function of the ascending reticular activating system or from a structural or metabolic lesion that is affecting both cortical hemispheres [1].

The most appropriate method of assessing the integrity of the ascending reticular activating system is to evaluate the status of the brainstem cranial nerves that are in close anatomic proximity to the ascending reticular activating system. In the midbrain this is limited to the third cranial nerve. Evaluating the third cranial nerve involves assessing the pupillary response to light and the extraocular movements controlled by this nerve (ability to move eyes medially and up and down: medial, superior, and inferior recti). When patients cannot voluntarily move their eyes, the oculocephalic reflex (doll's eyes) is tested or cold caloric reflexes are assessed. It is not possible to test the function of the fourth cranial nerve (intortion and nasal deviation of the eye) in a comatose patient. The integrity of the pons is evaluated by testing the fifth cranial nerve (afferent loop of the blink and nasal tickle response); the sixth cranial nerve (lateral eye movement: lateral rectus function); the seventh cranial nerve (efferent loop of blink reflex and facial muscle function); and the vestibular component of the eighth (afferent loop of the oculocephalic or cold caloric testing). Although lesions in the medulla do not cause coma, the medullary cranial nerves are routinely evaluated during the neurologic examination (gag and cough). Patients with impaired levels of consciousness including coma are still capable of exhibiting reflex motor functions. The most common test is the motor response to central pain. This is useful to localize a brainstem lesion below the red nucleus of the midbrain by extensor posturing (decerebrate) or above the midbrain by flexor posturing (decorticate). Patients able to localize painful stimuli are considered to have integrity of the motor system to a level above the diencephalons [1].

The experienced neurocritical care nurse uses these features of the neurologic examination to monitor for changes that may suggest new or evolving injury to specific CNS locations [63,64]. The most important change in the neurologic examination is a change in the patient's level of consciousness. A change in level of consciousness can range from a subtle change in the speed of response, to a profound and sudden inability to respond to stimuli. All changes in level of consciousness require investigation as to their cause. Other changes in the neurologic examination that require further investigation include focal motor change (inability to move an arm or leg); change in speech pattern (aphasia or dysarthria); and changes in cranial nerve reflexes. Changes in the neurologic examination can reflect a decrease in blood supply to areas of the brain. To recognize these potentially life-threatening cues accurately and promptly, the nurse must be able to detect patient changes from one examination to the next.

Changes in the patient's level of consciousness or neurologic level of function can be caused by local anatomic and systemic physiologic changes in the brain. Physical changes, such as edema and infarction, cause a dramatic change in the neurologic examination by direct injury to the brain tissue. Chemical changes, such as those seen with sedatives and opiates, can likewise cause a dramatic change in the neurologic examination, but these are reversible. Because these drugs may mask changes in the neurologic examination, the examination is most accurate when it is performed without the effects of these drugs.

When performing a neurologic examination on a patient who is receiving continuous intravenous sedation, a nurse is typically instructed to stop the infusion and perform the neurologic examination when the patient is awake. Several problems pertaining to definition arise in determining the construct of "awake"; what does awake mean and how does one determine adequacy of wakefulness to validate the results of a neurologic examination? Some methods of determining when the neurologic examination should be obtained after stopping the sedation infusion include watching for physical cues, such as patient movement, changing vital signs, and spontaneous neurologic function; repeating the examination until it is "as good as its going to get"; application of knowledge of the half-life of the sedative in use; and supplemental subjective assessment with objective information from the BIS index monitor.

Timing the neurologic examination based on subjective assessment

Critical care clinicians with refined assessment skills are often able to detect minor changes in their patients. Because of differences among patients, however, timing of the neurologic examination on the basis of visual cues can lead to misjudging the appropriate time for the neurologic examination, leading to misinterpretation of the findings. Poor interrater reliability between clinicians with varying levels of experience also contributes to timing issues for the neurologic examination when using subjective measures.

Timing the examination based on drug half-life

Although the effects of many medications, including sedatives, are often described in terms of their half-life, there are numerous factors that impact rates of metabolism, including hepatic function, renal clearance, and buildup in body fat stores. For this reason, it is neither practical nor reliable to make a determination of when to perform the neurologic examination based on drug half-life.

Timing the examination based on hemodynamic variables

Frequently, in the clinical setting there is a presumed relationship between a patient's hemodynamic response and relative level of sedation (ie, an increase in blood pressure and heart rate signal emergence from sedation). Flaishon and coworkers [65], however, demonstrated a lack of predictive relationship between vital signs and emergence from sedation. Changes in heart rate can be attributed to a variety of factors that are not related to emergence from sedation. Hypovolemia, infection, pain, hypotension, hypoxia, and activity can all contribute to an increased heart rate. Likewise, increased blood pressure may be related to changes in oxygen demand, intravascular fluid volume status, and electrolyte concentration, to name a few examples. A septic patient may be receiving a vasopressor to treat septic shock; an increase in blood pressure does not necessarily signal emergence from sedation, but may be a sign that the vasopressor is working.

The bispectral monitor

The BIS monitor was originally developed as an adjunctive tool for assessing level of consciousness during the intraoperative period. McCann and co-workers [12] found that BIS scores were a reliable indicator of patient movement to command during emergence from anesthesia for an intraoperative neurologic examination. In 2002, BIS monitors were first marketed to the ICU setting [66]. The BIS monitor provides a continuous digital reading of a signal-processed single-lead electroencephalogram waveform. The BIS scale varies from 0 to 100, with a score of zero corresponding to isoelectric activity and a score of 100 indicating full arousal. Higher BIS scores correlate with increased levels of arousal.

Interruption of sedation is necessary for neurologic assessment in the neurocritical care setting; however, daily interruptions in sedation may be useful in all areas of critical care [67]. Wake-up protocols have been associated with decreased mechanical ventilator days [6,68]. Because sedation titration should not occur solely on the basis of a single subjective assessment tool, using the BIS as an objective means of timing the sedation assessment the nurse is able to optimize accuracy of the neurologic examination and avoid severe, unnecessary, and potentially harmful decreases in levels of sedation.

Limitations of bispectral technology

The BIS monitor has several limitations that may preclude its use in every patient. The BIS monitor is placed on the forehead and monitors electrical activity in the frontal lobe. For patients with bilateral frontal lobe injury, or trauma patients in whom there is no space for the sensor, BIS monitoring is not practical. Recent data do suggest, however, that monitoring the occipital lobe may be an option when the frontal lobe is injured or otherwise unavailable [69]. Electromyographic interference from muscle activity can also affect signal-processed electroencephalogram of the BIS monitor. The most current algorithm uses a set of four leads to decrease the electromyographic artifact, but there are few studies demonstrating that this improves the reliability of the BIS values [70]. Certain medical therapeutics impact cerebral metabolic activity and may interfere with interpretation of BIS values. One study demonstrated that a decrease in muscle activity with chemical paralysis was associated with markedly lowered BIS values despite the subject being awake [71].

Although BIS values and ranges are used clinically, these are arbitrarily chosen and to date there have been no double-blinded randomized controlled trials that examine the efficacy of adjusting a sedative

medication to achieve a specific BIS value. One earlier investigation found only a moderate correlation between BIS values and subjective sedation assessment tools, concluding that "BIS is not suitable for monitoring the sedation in a heterogeneous group of surgical ICU patients" [72]. A criticism of the conclusion reached in this article is that although BIS was compared with the Sedation-Agitation Scale, modified observer's assessment of Alertness-Sedation Scale, and Ramsay Scale, cross-correlation between Ramsay Scale, Sedation-Agitation Scale, and observer's assessment of Alertness-Sedation Scale was not addressed [72]. Individual patient needs and response to medication impact the practitioner's decision to set a BIS goal. Further research is necessary to evaluate specific BIS values associated with best clinical outcomes.

Sedation interruption

Research support for a daily interruption in sedation is growing. The basic premise is that daily interruption in sedation allows for a reassessment of the patient's sedation requirements, prevents prolonged periods of oversedation, and decreases length of time on mechanical ventilatory support. Various authors have examined protocols requiring sedation interruption in the ICU setting. In one study the investigators [73] concluded that patients who received mechanical ventilatory support and continuous sedation experienced decreased length of stay and decreased time on mechanical ventilation resulting from a daily interruption in continuous sedation. Further support for a daily interruption was provided by a retrospective chart analysis that found a decrease in ICU complications and length of stay following daily interruption in continuous sedation. Several studies have found support for nurse-driven sedation protocols that include interruption and reassessment of continuous sedation [74,75]. Although studies have examined the usefulness of sedation interruption in yielding decreased length of stay, ventilator days, and complications, no studies have reported changes in important physiologic measures, such as intracranial pressure or hemodynamic alterations [67].

Timing the neurologic examination using bispectral technology

Recently, BIS monitoring has been gaining popularity in the ICU setting [13,76,77]. Growing evidence now supports the use of BIS monitoring as an adjunct to sedation assessment [5,77–81]. It is important to recognize, however, that this technology is not recommended as a solitary method of sedation assessment and should be combined with clinical assessments [70,80,82]. Typically, the BIS monitor is used for patients receiving continuous intravenous sedation with sedation goals being defined jointly in terms of a subjective scale, such as the Sedation-Agitation Scale or Ramsay Scale, and an objective BIS score. This combination of subjective and objective assessment has been associated with a reduced cost of sedation and decreased length of time on mechanical ventilation [5,13].

Nurses familiar with BIS monitoring are at a unique advantage when obtaining a neurologic examination on patients who are receiving continuous intravenous sedation. Instead of abruptly stopping the intravenous sedatives the nurse retains the option to decrease the infusion rate. Once the sedation is decreased, the nurse monitors for an increase in BIS values. As the BIS values increase, the patient experiences a return to consciousness. Decreasing, instead of stopping, the sedation while observing for an increase in BIS values may accomplish several goals. First, it allows the nurse to incorporate both subjective and objective data into determining when to perform the neurologic examination. Second, it markedly reduces the reliance on nonvalidated subjective clinical assessment parameters. Third, this reduces the risk of sudden changes in hemodynamic parameters associated with abrupt cessation of sedatives. Fourth, observing the trend in BIS values alerts the nurse that the patient is approaching consciousness, thereby reducing the risk of causing injury or harm, perhaps even decreasing the rate of unplanned self-extubation. By monitoring trended values and observing for values sustained greater than 80, nurses can use the BIS monitor to guide the timing of the assessment. BIS algorithms for processing the raw electroencephalogram signal can be used reliably to predict the level of arousal following a chemically induced sedation state [83].

Summary

The sedation-assessment conundrum arises from the conflict between two opposing goals: to maintain a safe and comfortable environment for the patient through the use of sedation, and the need for accurate neurologic evaluation that reflects the patient's best possible effort. Planned interruption of continuous

intravenous sedation is a necessary part of routine nursing practice in the neuroscience critical care unit. The use of BIS monitoring as an adjunctive tool for sedation assessment to facilitate planned interruption in sedation is helpful in achieving a valid neurologic assessment.

Critical care nurses are highly proficient at integrating specialized knowledge, skills, and technology into practice. Sandelowski [84] writes, "As the primary machine tenders in health care, nurses often acquire an understanding of how to apply, operate, and interpret the products of devices that becomes an integral part of the tacit know-how of clinical practice." Knowing how and when to place faith in technology, and to find the balance between objective and subjective assessment, allows for solutions to the sedation–neurologic assessment conundrum.

References

[1] Blumenfeld H. Neuroanatomy through clinical cases. Sunderland (MA): Sinauer; 2002.

[2] Greenberg MS. Handbook of neurosurgery. 5th edition. Lakeland (FL): Thieme; 2001.

[3] Arbour R. Continuous nervous system monitoring, EEG, the bispectral index, and neuromuscular transmission. AACN Clin Issues 2003;14:185–207.

[4] Mirski MA, Muffelman B, Ulatowski JA, et al. Sedation for the critically ill neurologic patient. Crit Care Med 1995;23:2038–53.

[5] Olson DM, Chioffi SM, Macy GE, et al. Potential benefits of bispectral index monitoring in critical care: a case study. Crit Care Nurse 2003;23:45–52.

[6] Burchardi H. Aims of sedation/analgesia. Minerva Anestesiol 2004;70:137–43.

[7] Jacobi J, Fraser GL, Coursin DB, et al. Clinical practice guidelines for the sustained use of sedatives and analgesics in the critically ill adult. Crit Care Med 2002;30:119–41.

[8] Murdoch S, Cohen A. Intensive care sedation: a review of current British practice. Intensive Care Med 2000; 26:922–8.

[9] Young C, Knudsen N, Hilton A, et al. Sedation in the intensive care unit. Crit Care Med 2000;28:854–66.

[10] Dennis LJ, Mayer SA. Diagnosis and management of increased intracranial pressure. Neurol India 2001; 49(Suppl 1):S37–50.

[11] Alspach J. American Association of Critical-Care Nurses: core curriculum for critical care nursing. 5th edition. Philadelphia: WB Saunders; 1998.

[12] McCann ME, Brustowicz RM, Bacsik J, et al. The bispectral index and explicit recall during the intraoperative wake-up test for scoliosis surgery. Anesth Analg 2002;94:1474–8.

[13] Olson DM, Cheek DJ, Morgenlander JC. The impact

of bispectral index monitoring on rates of propofol administration. AACN Clin Issues 2004;15:63–73.

[14] Berkenbosch JW, Fichter CR, Tobias JD. The correlation of the bispectral index monitor with clinical sedation scores during mechanical ventilation in the pediatric intensive care unit. Anesth Analg 2002;94: 506–11.

[15] Avramov MN, White PF. Methods for monitoring the level of sedation. Crit Care Clin 1995;11:803–26.

[16] Schmidlin D, Hager P, Schmid ER. Monitoring level of sedation with bispectral EEG analysis: comparison between hypothermic and normothermic cardiopulmonary bypass. Br J Anaesth 2001;86:769–76.

[17] Devlin JW, Fraser GL, Kanji S, et al. Sedation assessment in critically ill adults. Ann Pharmacother 2001;35:1624–32.

[18] Ramsay MA, Savege TM, Simpson BR, et al. Controlled sedation with alphaxalone-alphadolone. BMJ 1974;2:656–9.

[19] Riker RR, Picard JT, Fraser GL. Prospective evaluation of the sedation-agitation scale for adult critically ill patients. Crit Care Med 1999;27:1325–9.

[20] Riker RR, Fraser GL, Simmons LE, et al. Validating the sedation-agitation scale with the bispectral index and visual analog scale in adult ICU patients after cardiac surgery. Intensive Care Med 2001;27: 853–8.

[21] Sessler CN, Gosnell MS, Grap MJ, et al. The Richmond agitation-sedation scale: validity and reliability in adult intensive care unit patients. Am J Respir Crit Care Med 2002;166:1338–44.

[22] de Lemos J, Tweeddale M, Chittock D. Measuring quality of sedation in adult mechanically ventilated critically ill patients: the Vancouver Interaction and Calmness Scale. Sedation Focus Group. J Clin Epidemiol 2000;53:908–19.

[23] Chernik DA, Gillings D, Laine H, et al. Validity and reliability of the Observer's Assessment of Alertness/ Sedation Scale: study with intravenous midazolam. J Clin Psychopharmacol 1990;10:244–51.

[24] Muller-Busch HC, Andres I, Jehser T. Sedation in palliative care: a critical analysis of 7 years experience. BMC Palliat Care 2003;2:2.

[25] Braun TC, Hagen NA, Clark T. Development of a clinical practice guideline for palliative sedation. J Palliat Med 2003;6:345–50.

[26] Magarey JM. Sedation of adult critically ill ventilated patients in intensive care units: a national survey. Aust Crit Care 1997;10:90–3.

[27] Rodrigues Jr GR, do Amaral JL. Influence of sedation on morbidity and mortality in the intensive care unit. Sao Paulo Med J 2004;122:8–11.

[28] Park G, Coursin D, Ely EW, et al. Commentary: balancing sedation and analgesia in the critically ill. Crit Care Clin 2001;17:1015–27.

[29] Guin PR, Freudenberger K. The elderly neuroscience patient: implications for the critical care nurse. AACN Clin Issues Crit Care Nurs 1992;3:98–105.

[30] Vasile B, Rasulo F, Candiani A, et al. The pathophysiology of propofol infusion syndrome: a simple name for a complex syndrome. Intensive Care Med 2003; 29:1417–25.

[31] Valente JF, Anderson GL, Branson RD, et al. Disadvantages of prolonged propofol sedation in the critical care unit. Crit Care Med 1994;22:710–2.

[32] Cannon ML, Glazier SS, Bauman LA. Metabolic acidosis, rhabdomyolysis, and cardiovascular collapse after prolonged propofol infusion. J Neurosurg 2001; 95:1053–6.

[33] de Wit M, Epstein SK. Administration of sedatives and level of sedation: comparative evaluation via the sedation-agitation scale and the bispectral index. Am J Crit Care 2003;12:343–8.

[34] Boulain T. Unplanned extubations in the adult intensive care unit: a prospective multicenter study. Association des Reanimateurs du Centre-Ouest. Am J Respir Crit Care Med 1998;157(4 Pt 1):1131–7.

[35] Tung A, Tadimeti L, Caruana-Montaldo B, et al. The relationship of sedation to deliberate self-extubation. J Clin Anesth 2001;13:24–9.

[36] Cheng EY. Recall in the sedated ICU patient. J Clin Anesth 1996;8:675–8.

[37] Wagner BK, Zavotsky KE, Sweeney JB, et al. Patient recall of therapeutic paralysis in a surgical critical care unit. Pharmacotherapy 1998;18:358–63.

[38] Ostermann ME, Keenan SP, Seiferling RA, et al. Sedation in the intensive care unit: a systematic review. JAMA 2000;283:1451–9.

[39] Rhoney DH, Murry KR. National survey on the use of sedatives and neuromuscular blocking agents in the pediatric intensive care unit. Pediatr Crit Care Med 2002;3:129–33.

[40] Gross JB, Bailey PL, Connis RT, et al. Practice guidelines for sedation and analgesia by non-anesthesiologists: an updated report by the American Society of Anesthesiologists task force on sedation and analgesia by non-anesthesiologists. Anesthesiology 2002;96:1004–17.

[41] Donnelly AJ, Golembiewski JA. Perioperative care. In: Koda-Kimble MA, Young LY, Kradjan WA, editors. Applied therapeutics: the clinical use of drugs. 7th edition. Baltimore: Lippincott Williams & Wilkins; 2001. p. 8.1–8.42.

[42] Kandel ER, Schwartz JH, Jessell TM. Principles of neural science. 4th edition. New York: McGraw-Hill Health Professions Division; 2000.

[43] Bayat A, Arscott G. Continuous intravenous versus bolus parenteral midazolam: a safe technique for conscious sedation in plastic surgery. Br J Plast Surg 2003;56:272–5.

[44] Deem S. Useful information about the pharmacokinetics and pharmacodynamics of midazolam and lorazepam. Anesthesiology 2002;97:522 [author reply: 522–3].

[45] Miller RD, Reves JG. Anesthesia. Philadelphia: Churchill Livingstone; 2000.

[46] Ronan KP, Gallagher TJ, George B, et al. Comparison of propofol and midazolam for sedation in

intensive care unit patients. Crit Care Med 1995;23:
286 – 93.

[47] McMurray TJ, Collier PS, Carson IW, et al. Propofol
sedation after open heart surgery: a clinical and
pharmacokinetic study. Anaesthesia 1990;45:322 – 6.

[48] Schuttler J, Ihmsen H. Population pharmacokinetics of
propofol: a multicenter study. Anesthesiology 2000;92:
727 – 38.

[49] Frenkel C, Schuttler J, Ihmsen H, et al. Pharmacokinetics and pharmacodynamics of propofol/alfentanil
infusions for sedation in ICU patients. Intensive Care
Med 1995;21:981 – 8.

[50] Barrientos-Vega R, Mar Sanchez-Soria M, Morales-
Garcia C, et al. Prolonged sedation of critically ill
patients with midazolam or propofol: impact on
weaning and costs. Crit Care Med 1997;25:33 – 40.

[51] Cecil RL, Goldman L, Bennett JC. Cecil textbook
of medicine. 21st edition. Philadelphia: WB Saunders; 2000.

[52] Hvidberg EF, Dam M. Clinical pharmacokinetics of
anticonvulsants. Clin Pharmacokinet 1976;1:161 – 88.

[53] Ehrnebo M. Pharmacokinetics and distribution properties of pentobarbital in humans following oral and
intravenous administration. J Pharm Sci 1974;63:
1114 – 8.

[54] Millgate AG, Pogson BJ, Wilson IW, et al. Analgesia:
morphine-pathway block in top1 poppies. Nature 2004;
431:413 – 4.

[55] Ford MD. Clinical toxicology. Philadelphia: WB Saunders; 2001.

[56] Lugo RA, Kern SE. Clinical pharmacokinetics of
morphine. J Pain Palliat Care Pharmacother 2002;16:
5 – 18.

[57] Kharasch ED, Hoffer C, Whittington D. Influence of
age on the pharmacokinetics and pharmacodynamics
of oral transmucosal fentanyl citrate. Anesthesiology
2004;101:738 – 43.

[58] Sindrup SH, Brosen K. The pharmacogenetics of codeine hypoalgesia. Pharmacogenetics 1995;5:335 – 46.

[59] Kirby GW. Biosynthesis of the morphine alkaloids.
Science 1967;155:170 – 3.

[60] Venn RM, Grounds RM. Comparison between dexmedetomidine and propofol for sedation in the intensive
care unit: patient and clinician perceptions. Br J
Anaesth 2001;87:684 – 90.

[61] Ebert T, Maze M. Dexmedetomidine: another arrow
for the clinician's quiver. Anesthesiology 2004;101:
568 – 70.

[62] Teasdale G, Jennett B. Assessment of coma and impaired consciousness: a practical scale. Lancet 1974;2:
81 – 4.

[63] Adomat R, Hicks C. Measuring nursing workload in
intensive care: an observational study using closed
circuit video cameras. J Adv Nurs 2003;42:402 – 12.

[64] Benner P. From novice to expert: excellence and power
in clinical nursing practice. Menlo Park (CA): Addi-
son-Wesley, Nursing Division; 1984.

[65] Flaishon R, Windsor A, Sigl J, et al. Recovery of
consciousness after thiopental or propofol: bispectral

index and isolated forearm technique. Anesthesiology
1997;86:613 – 9.

[66] Aspect Medical Systems. Company information about
Aspect Company timeline. Available at: http://www.
aspectms.com. Accessed November 2004.

[67] Schweickert WD, Gehlbach BK, Pohlman AS, et al.
Daily interruption of sedative infusions and complications of critical illness in mechanically ventilated
patients. Crit Care Med 2004;32:1272 – 6.

[68] MacIntyre NR. Evidence-based ventilator weaning and
discontinuation. Respir Care 2004;49:830 – 6.

[69] Shiraishi T, Uchino H, Sagara T, et al. A comparison of
frontal and occipital bispectral index values obtained
during neurosurgical procedures. Anesth Analg 2004;
98:1773 – 5.

[70] Vivien B, Di Maria S, Ouattara A, et al. Over-
estimation of bispectral index in sedated intensive care
unit patients revealed by administration of muscle
relaxant. Anesthesiology 2003;99:9 – 17.

[71] Messner M, Beese U, Romstock J, et al. The bispectral
index declines during neuromuscular block in fully
awake persons. Anesth Analg 2003;97:488 – 91.

[72] Frenzel D, Greim CA, Sommer C, et al. Is the
bispectral index appropriate for monitoring the sedation level of mechanically ventilated surgical ICU
patients? Intensive Care Med 2002;28:178 – 83.

[73] Kress JP, Pohlman AS, O'Connor MF, et al. Daily
interruption of sedative infusions in critically ill
patients undergoing mechanical ventilation. N Engl J
Med 2000;342:1471 – 7.

[74] Kollef MH, Levy NT, Ahrens TS, et al. The use of
continuous i.v. sedation is associated with prolongation of mechanical ventilation. Chest 1998;114:
541 – 8.

[75] Brook AD, Ahrens TS, Schaiff R, et al. Effect of a
nursing-implemented sedation protocol on the duration
of mechanical ventilation. Crit Care Med 1999;27:
2609 – 15.

[76] Simmons LE, Riker RR, Prato BS, et al. Assessing sedation during intensive care unit mechanical ventilation with the bispectral index and the
sedation-agitation scale. Crit Care Med 1999;27:
1499 – 504.

[77] Hilbish C. Bispectral index monitoring in the neu-
rointensive care unit. J Neurosci Nurs 2003;35:
336 – 8.

[78] Arbour RB. Using the bispectral index to assess
arousal response in a patient with neuromuscular
blockade. Am J Crit Care 2000;9:383 – 7.

[79] Kaplan LJ, Bailey H. Bispectral index (BIS) monitoring of ICU patients on continuous infusion of sedatives
and paralytics reduces sedative drug utilization and
cost. Crit Care Med 2000;4:S110.

[80] Mondello E, Siliotti R, Noto G, et al. Bispectral index in ICU: correlation with Ramsay score on assessment of sedation level. J Clin Monit Comput 2002;17:
271 – 7.

[81] Triltsch AE, Welte M, von Homeyer P, et al. Bispectral
index-guided sedation with dexmedetomidine in inten-

sive care: a prospective, randomized, double blind, placebo-controlled phase II study. Crit Care Med 2002; 30:1007–14.

[82] Riess ML, Graefe UA, Goeters C, et al. Sedation assessment in critically ill patients with bispectral index. Eur J Anaesthesiol 2002;19:18–22.

[83] Billard V, Gambus PL, Chamoun N, et al. A comparison of spectral edge, delta power, and bispec-

tral index as EEG measures of alfentanil, propofol, and midazolam drug effect. Clin Pharmacol Ther 1997; 61:45–58.

[84] Sandelowski M. Knowing and forgetting: the challenge of technology for a reflexive practice science of nursing. In: Thorne SE, Hayes VE, editors. Nursing praxis knowledge and action. Thousand Oaks (CA): Sage Publications; 1997. p. 69–85.

ELSEVIER
SAUNDERS

Crit Care Nurs Clin N Am 17 (2005) 269 – 277

CRITICAL CARE
NURSING CLINICS
OF NORTH AMERICA

Obstructive Sleep Apnea and Modifications in Sedation

Cheryl Kabeli, FNP

Department of Cardiology, Champlain Valley Physicians Hospital, 75 Beekman Street, Plattsburgh, NY 12901, USA

Sleep disorders have been a neglected aspect of medicine, and all too often remain undetected. Sleep occupies approximately one third of each person's lifetime, but its impact on health and medical conditions remains largely unrecognized. The prevalence of obstructive sleep apnea (OSA) in middle age is 2% for women and 4% for men [1]. In the clinical setting, OSA is diagnosed in an estimated 20% of patients; however, it may go unreported [2]. This leaves a large portion of the population with under-diagnosed or undiagnosed OSA.

Physicians and nurses have recognized an increase in morbidity and mortality in patients with OSA when they are administered anesthesia in conjunction with sedation. There are few reports of sedation alone and OSA; most studies have been in relation to anesthesia, surgery, patient-controlled analgesia, and sleep-disordered breathing.

Basic mechanisms of sleep

Sleep is divided into two phases. The first is rapid eye movement (REM) and is most often associated with vivid dreaming and high levels of brain activity. The second phase of sleep is non-REM, and is usually associated with reduced neuronal activity. In this stage the content is typically nonvisual and consists of ruminative thought [3].

The first REM period usually occurs approximately 90 to 120 minutes after the onset of sleep. In REM sleep there is suppression of muscle tone

(typically measured in the chin muscle on sleep studies) and the presence of REMs [3]. The first episode is short. After the first REM episode, the stages of the sleep cycle are repeated and non-REM sleep occurs. Approximately 90 minutes after the start of the first REM period, another REM cycle begins. This continuous cycling persists throughout the night. A sleep cycle is approximately 90 minutes and the duration of each REM sleep episode after the first is approximately 30 minutes (Table 1) [3].

The physiologic mechanisms responsible for initiating and terminating sleep and establishing it in its various forms can all become disorganized, attenuated, or exaggerated [4]. These alterations are the basis of sleep disorders. There are generally three different types of apnea. The first is central sleep apnea resulting from withdrawal of central drive, which is apnea without ventilatory effort. This occurs in a small portion of the population. The second type is OSA, characterized by repeated episodes of upper airway closure at sleep [4,5]. This prevents air from entering the lungs, thereby interrupting the continuous exchange of gas in the lungs. During these periods, hypoxemia is the major stimuli for arousal. Carbon dioxide does not rise to a significant level while arterial oxygen partial pressure falls rapidly [5,6]. After arousal, the patient usually falls asleep quickly with no awareness of the events. These multiple episodes of apnea reduce arterial oxygen saturation to less then 80% [6–8]. It is when this happens that accompanying cardiac arrhythmias occur [8]. The third type of sleep apnea is mixed apnea, a combination of central and OSA. It involves brief periods of central apnea followed by longer periods of OSA. There is initially no ventilatory effort, but an OSA pattern is evident when effort resumes [7,8].

E-mail address: corishrn@yahoo.com

Table 1
Stages of sleep

Stage	Action
Wakefulness	Body prepares for sleep. Muscles begin to relax. Eye movement slows to a roll.
Stage 1	May last for 5–10 min. Eyes are closed, but if aroused, may feel as if he or she has not slept.
Stage 2	Period of light sleep. Spontaneous periods of muscle tone mixed with periods of muscle relaxation. Heart rate slows. Body temperature decreases. Body prepares to enter deep sleep. Up to 65% of sleep is spent in this stage
Stage 3 and 4	Deep stages of sleep. Stage 4 more intense. Known as slow wave or delta sleep. EMG shows a pattern of deep sleep and rhythmic continuity.
Non-REM sleep	Comprises stage 1–4 and lasts from 90–120 min, each stage lasting anywhere from 5–15 min.
REM (stage 5)	Occurs 90 min after sleep onset. Characteristic rapid eye movements. Heart rate and respiration speed up and become more erratic. Intense dreaming occurs. The first period of REM typically lasts 10 min, the final one lasting 1 h.

Cessation of airflow for 10 seconds has been widely but arbitrarily used as a definition of apnea [9]. Hypopneas is defined as a >50% decrease in airflow or a <50% decrease in airflow associated with a change in oxygen saturations of at least 3% or an electroencephalogram arousal [4,9]. The apnea plus hypopnea index is the most commonly used measure of sleep-disordered breathing. It is the sum of apnea plus hypopnea episodes that a person has in an overnight sleep study divided by the total sleep time in hours (Box 1). The total number helps to determine the severity of the sleep disorder. Respiratory effort-related arousal is defined as a sequence of breaths characterized by increasing respiratory effort leading to an arousal from sleep that does not meet criteria for an apnea or hypopnea. Most sleep-disordered breathing falls into this category.

Respiratory-induced arousals minimize the duration and extent of apneas and hypoxia in the short-term, but the sleep fragmentation reduces ventilatory drive and both the strength and the endurance of the respiratory muscles in the upper airway and chest wall [4]. The effects on the respiratory drive are reversible and improve once sleep fragmentation is relieved, but are exacerbated by sedation and alcohol [10–12].

Assessment

The gold standard for diagnosing and staging the severity of sleep apnea is a standard overnight polysomnography. Electrodes are applied to the limbs and movement is recorded along with the electrophysiologic signals. Signals include a video recording, an electroencephalogram with two leads, electromyography, electro-oculography, respiratory signals from airflow measurements from nasal pressure, nasal temperature, expired carbon dioxide, ventilation from thoracoabdominal movements or nasal pressure, oxygenation levels, and possible esophageal balloon pressures [13,14]. Other signals include an electrocardiogram tracing during sleep, pulse rate, position, esophageal pH, and video recording.

Obtaining a thorough sleep history and a medical history and physical can help identify patients who are at high risk (Box 2). The physical examination should include documentation of the blood pressure; body mass index; neck circumference (especially short and fat neck); evidence for vascular disease; and any abnormalities of the upper airway. Upper airway abnormalities of concern include the presence of nasal polyps, septal deviation, previous nasal fractures, crowed pharynx, presence of macroglossia; uvula shape, size, length, and movement during phonation; and the presence of inflammation of any of the upper airway structures [4,15]. The uvula, although rarely responsible for snoring, may be red, inflamed, elongated, and unable to lift off the base of the tongue during phonation because of snoring.

There are many subjective evaluation tools that patients can complete to help identify this problem.

Multiple Sleep Latency Test
Stanford Sleepiness Scale
Epworth Sleepiness Scale
Pittsburgh Sleep Quality Index
Sleep logs, diaries, and charts
Visual Analog and Rating Scale

Box 1. Apnea plus hypopnea index criteria

Normal <5
Mild 5 to 15
Moderate 15 to 30
Severe >30

Sleep apnea syndrome: apnea plus hypopnea index of >5 with symptoms.

Box 2. Sleep history assessment

- Description of the sleep problem
  (ie, nature, severity, duration, signs
  and symptoms, effect)
- Usual sleep pattern
- Recent changes in sleep pattern
- Bedtime routine
- Sleep environment
- Diet, alcohol intake
- Symptoms during waking hours
- Use of medication (over-the-counter,
  prescription, sleeping pills)
- Concurrent physical illness
- Recent life events
- Current emotional and mental status

*Symptoms associated with
sleep-disordered breathing*

- Persistent snoring
- Excessive daytime sleepiness
- Apneas (noted by bed partner)
- Gastrointestinal reflux disease
- Personality changes
- Mood swings
- Restless sleep
- Morning headaches
- Impotence
- Reduced ability to concentrate
- Choking sensations

The Epworth Sleepiness Scale is the most commonly used scale in the literature as a subjective measurement of sleepiness. The Epworth Sleepiness Scale is used to determine the level of daytime sleepiness (Fig. 1). It is used to distinguish primary snoring from OSA. The Epworth Sleepiness Scale has a possible score range of 0 to 24. A total score of 10 or more suggests further evaluation is needed to determine the cause of excessive sleepiness or determine if an underlying sleep disorder may be present [16].

A history should be sought of previous surgery or trauma to the upper airways (any site between the nose and the larynx) because the compliance of the airways may be affected. A family predisposition to snoring has been described, and many who snore admit to other family members having a history of snoring. A sleep history assessment can be obtained

from both the patient and their bed partner. A thorough medical history is needed to determine comorbid conditions.

Upper airway compliance and loss of upper airway muscle activity

The upper airway is more collapsible in individuals with OSA than in patients without OSA because of a combination of neurologic and mechanical factors [17,18]. Airway compliance is influenced by a combination of features, such as tissue damage and edema [19]. These can be caused from trauma of OSA and snoring. Factors that predispose individuals to OSA from upper airway resistance are sleep deprivation and fragmentation, benzodiazepines, alcohol, general anesthesia, and ventilatory support [20].

Benzodiazepines increase the level of inspiratory effort required to cause arousal at the end of an OSA through their central nervous system depressant activity [4]. They may also increase the degree of muscle relaxation in the upper airway.

Alcohol has similar effects. The decrease in arousability prolongs the apneic period. This impairs the postapnea hyperventilation so that the rate of oxygen resaturation is slower. Alcohol also increases the nasal airflow resistance by causing hyperemia of the nasal mucosa [4,12]. General anesthesia causes the central control of the upper airway to be altered so that the muscles lose their activity. Ventilatory support causes the loss of the normal sequence of muscle contraction in which the upper airway muscles are activated before the chest wall muscles [21].

Pharmacology

The main use of benzodiazepines and hypnotics is for promoting sleep and sedation. The aim of treatment should not be simply to increase the quality and duration of sleep and sedation, but also to prevent any residual sleepiness the next day and avoid other features of central nervous system depression [22].

Benzodiazepines

These are rapidly absorbed from the gastrointestinal tract, although this is slowed by food and

0 = no chance of dozing
1 = slight chance of dozing
2 = moderate chance of dozing
3 = high chance of dozing

SITUATION	CHANCE OF DOZING
Sitting and reading	
Watching TV	
Sitting inactive in a public place (E.G. a theater or a meeting)	
As a passenger in a car for an hour without a break	
Lying down to rest in the afternoon when circumstances permit	
Sitting and talking to someone	
Sitting quietly after a lunch without alcohol	
In a car, while stopped for a few minutes in traffic	

Fig. 1. Epworth Sleepiness Scale.

antacids. A clinical effect is apparent with most of these drugs within 1 hour and the peak plasma level is usually reached between 1 and 3 hours after ingestion. Some benzodiazepines, such as triazolam and midazolam, have few active metabolites but diazepam is metabolized to desmethyldiazepam, which is active and has a half-life of 50 to 100 hours [23]. This metabolite is not produced by lorazepam or oxazepam.

Benzodiazepines in low doses have a sedative effect and in higher doses induce sleep (Table 2). They increase total sleep time, shorten sleep latency, decrease the number of awakenings, and provide a sense of deep and refreshing sleep [4,22]. REM sleep latency is prolonged, the duration of REM sleep is reduced, there are fewer eye movements, and less dreaming during REM sleep, except with short-acting drugs, such as triazolam, which cause a rebound in REM sleep late in the night [4]. Sleep is consolidated in that there are sleep-stage transitions, but the duration of stage 3 and 4 non-REM sleep is reduced in parallel with that of REM sleep [4]. The duration of stage 2 sleep increases. Withdrawal of benzodiazepines leads to REM sleep rebound, which may be associated with vivid dreams and nightmares for several weeks.

Table 2
Commonly used benzodiazepines and hypnotics for sleep

Drug	Dose (mg)	Effect of single dose on sleep	Effect of regular dose in daytime	Uses
Triazolam	0.125–25	Short acting	None	Brief daytime and nocturnal sleep, DIS
Midazolam	1–5	Short acting	None	DIS
Diazepam	2–10	Short acting	Sedation	Transient DIS, DMS, and EMW with anxiety
Temazepam	7.5–30	Intermediate	Mild sedation	DIS, DMS
Oxazepam	10–30	Intermediate	None	DMS, EMW with anxiety
Clonazepam	0.25–0.5	Long acting	Sedation	DMS, EMW with anxiety
Zolpidem	5–10	Short acting	None	DIS
Zaleplon	5–10	Short acting	None	DIS, DMS

Abbreviations: DIS, difficulty in initiating sleep; DMS, difficulty in maintaining sleep; EMW, early morning awakening.

Daytime sedation is most pronounced with benzodiazepines with a long duration of action, particularly if the drugs are given for prolonged periods and in high doses. The degree of sedation during the day also depends on the balance between the improvement in sleep quality and the "hangover" effect of continuous sedation [4]. Termination of benzodiazepines may lead to recurrence or even temporary worsening of the original symptoms. A specific withdrawal syndrome may also appear and is characterized by disturbed sleep, vivid dreams, and nightmares associated with an increase in REM sleep and in stage 3 and 4 non-REM sleep [4,23]. The problem of rebound insomnia occurs either during each night of treatment or withdrawal of regular treatment. Rebound insomnia during treatment is associated with short-acting drugs, which do not accumulate in the body.

Nonbenzodiazepines and hypnotics

Two commonly prescribed drugs for both inpatients and outpatients are zolpidem and zaleplon. These drugs at appropriate prescribed doses have little effect on sleep architecture in contrast to the benzodiazepines [24]. The sedative properties of both these drugs are much more pronounced then their anxiolytic or muscle relaxing properties.

Zolpidem, with its short duration of action, occasionally leads to rebound insomnia later in the night. It rarely causes daytime sedation because of its short duration of action, but can lead to nausea, vomiting, diarrhea, headaches, and dizziness. Zolpidem seems to be as effective a hypnotic as the benzodiazepines [24]. Its indications are similar to this group of drugs.

Zaleplon is a very short acting hypnotic whose main indications are in treating difficulty in initiating sleep. This can be used for night shift workers who wish to sleep during the day. Zaleplon has a dose-related effect in reducing sleep latency, but because of its short duration of action it does not increase the total sleep time or decrease the number of awakenings. Rebound insomnia later in the night is uncommon.

Barbiturates

Barbiturates may cause sedation, sleep, anesthesia, and even death according to the dose, age, individual susceptibility, and interaction with other drugs [23]. They have a similar effect on sleep to the benzodiazepines in that they reduce the sleep latency and the duration of REM sleep, and REM sleep latency increases. The duration of stage 2 non-REM sleep is increased, but stage 3 and 4 non-REM sleep become shorter and the number of arousals is reduced [4]. Withdrawal of barbiturates after prolonged use leads to REM sleep rebound with nightmare and rebound insomnia. Patients are known to develop tolerance to these drugs and have a high risk for dependence.

Alcohol

Alcohol is an anxiolytic and a weak hypnotic. It increases the total sleep time, reduces sleep latency, reduces the latency before stage 3 and 4 non-REM sleep, increases their duration, and suppresses REM sleep [11,12]. It is short acting so that as the blood alcohol level falls during the night REM sleep rebound occurs. This often occurs with vivid dreams, loss of non-REM sleep, and frequent awakenings.

High doses may also reduce the duration of stage 3 and 4 non-REM sleep and its diuretic effects causes awakening from sleep [10,12]. It also induces OSA, which leads to sleep fragmentation. Its general depressant effects can increase the duration of periods of apnea, worsening a pre-existing OSA [10,12]. The pharmacologic effects of alcohol are combined with episodes of partial withdrawal and dehydration, which leads to difficulty in maintaining sleep. Frequent sleep-stage shifts and arousals lead to both insomnia and excessive daytime sleepiness. Acute withdrawal of alcohol after long-term consumption causes REM sleep rebound with a short REM latency, a reduction in stage 3 and 4 non-REM sleep, and sleep fragmentation with an increase in the number of sleep-stage shifts and awakenings. This may lead to reinitiation of alcohol intake in the acute care setting, but if abstinence can be maintained for about 2 weeks these symptoms gradually improve. The sleep pattern may remain abnormal with frequent awakenings for up to 2 years [4].

Opioids

Opioids are agents that induce systemic analgesia, some anxiolysis, and mild sedation. They do not induce amnesia of any significance. They act by binding to specific opioid receptors in the central nervous system and spinal cord. Respiratory depression is the most serious side effect of opioids when administering them for sedation. At low doses, respiratory tidal volume is unaffected and only respiratory rate is decreased. At increasing doses, both tidal volume and respiratory rate are affected. Irregularities of respiratory pattern are associated with opioid analgesia after major operation and may contribute to patient hypoxia, apneas, and cardiovascular deterioration [8,19,24,25]. Opioids reduce total sleep time, increase sleep latency, and increase the number of arousals. They also lead to sleep fragmentation, reduce the duration of REM sleep, and increase stage 2, but decrease stage 3 and 4 non-REM sleep. Withdrawal of opioids lead to rebound insomnia, rebound increase in REM sleep, and to a lesser extent a rebound increase in stage 3 and 4 non-REM sleep for up to several days [4].

Morphine is the oldest and most established agent for systemic analgesia. Given intravenously, it has a rapid onset and duration of action of as long as 3 to 4 hours. It can be given intramuscularly, but it has a delayed onset and a smaller analgesic effect in this case. Adverse effects include hypotension, which is partly mediated by histamine release. Slower rates of administration minimize this effect. Respiratory depression can occur; it is uncommon at typical doses, but increases with coadministration of sedative agents. Fentanyl is a potent synthetic opioid with some characteristics that warrant its use outside the operating room. It has short duration of action (as long as $1-2$ hours) and minimal cardiovascular effects, such as hypotension. If given appropriately, respiratory depression is uncommon, but this effect lasts longer than its analgesic effect. It is the preferred drug for analgesia in short procedures and is an alternative to morphine in cases of trauma in which hemodynamic compromise may be problematic.

Anesthesia and sleep-disordered breathing

Current knowledge strongly suggests that anesthetic, sedation, and analgesic agents aggravate or precipitate OSA. This is done by decreasing pharyngeal tone; depressing ventilatory responses to hypoxia and hypercapnia; and inhibiting arousal responses to obstruction, hypoxia, and hypercapnia [21]. Anesthetics and narcotic agents also impair normal arousal mechanisms, thereby worsening apnea severity [21]. It has also been noted that even in healthy patients, anesthetic and analgesia can develop postoperative obstructions [19,26]. These later effects frequently result in varying degrees of central respiratory depression. Jain and Dhand [19] state sedation and anesthesia reduce functional residual capacity and predispose the patient to atelectasis.

A variety of surgical factors are also contributory. Surgery involving the upper airway carries the risk of postoperative swelling that can worsen or precipitate obstruction [19]. Surgery of the thorax and upper abdomen compromises ventilatory function [27], potentially compounding the effects of any OSA or central mediated hypoventilation that might occur postoperatively [19,27]. Rennotte and coworkers [28] reported on 16 adult patients with documented OSA undergoing various types of surgical procedures, including coronary artery bypass surgery. Anesthesia was administered with the usual type of drug for each type of surgery. Postoperative opioid analgesia and sedation were not restricted. One patient with previously diagnosed but untreated OSA died after various complications, including respiratory arrest in the hospital bed. Another patient experienced serious postoperative complications, including failed extubation, until treatment for OSA with nasal continuous positive airway pressure was instituted, and then made an uneventful recovery.

A clinical suspicion of sleep apnea may first develop at the preadmission testing area or preoperative holding area before surgery. A risk assessment tool may be helpful to categorize these patients before induction (Table 3). Intraoperatively, a patient might present with a difficult intubation by anesthesia personnel. Hiremath and coworkers [29] showed that patients in whom the trachea was difficult to intubate were at increased risk for OSA. The study noted that anatomic changes seem to be responsible for difficulty in intubation. While awake, patients were able to compensate with positional changes of the upper airway. The compensation may be lost with muscle relaxation during sleep or when under the influence of sedatives, neuromuscular blockade, or anesthetic agents [30]. Postoperative recovery with snoring further warrants investigation. Obesity (body

Table 3
Sleep apnea risk assessment tool

High risk	Low risk
Male	No snoring
Body mass index > 25 kg/m^2	Premenopausal
Neck circumference	Thin
>17 in in men	
>16 in in women	
Snoring or gasping (noted by bed partner)	
Excessive daytime sleepiness	
Hypertension	

Adapted from Meoli AL, Rosen C, Kristo D, et al. Upper airway management of the adult patient with obstructive sleep apnea in the perioperative period avoiding complications. Sleep 2003;26:1060–5.

mass index >30), especially with a large neck circumference, has a positive correlation with severe OSA, because these conditions involve extensive soft tissue enlargement of the upper airway [9,31].

Anesthesia and airway conditions are as important in children as adults. Waters and coworkers [25] studied children with OSA in the common clinical environment of inhaled anesthesia. They showed fentanyl led to central apnea requiring respiratory support in 46% of children with OSA and concluded that children with OSA are particularly sensitive to respiratory depression caused by opiates.

The anesthetic management plan should be determined by the severity of sleep apnea, how it has been managed before anesthesia, the surgical procedure, and the postoperative analgesia needed for patient comfort. This information should be shared with all staff that is caring for the patient. The use of premedication in patients with OSA is controversial [8,9,28]. Appropriate monitoring with oxygen saturation and visual observation is essential. An unsupervised holding area is inappropriate for a premedicated sleep apnea patient. An intravenous catheter should be placed and reversal agents readily available.

Herder and coworkers [9] suggest preoperative sedation with benzodiazepines about 45 minutes before the induction of general anesthesia has an anticonvulsive and muscular relaxing effect on the upper airway, causing an appreciable reduction of the pharyngeal space. Consequently, a higher risk of preoperative phases of hypopneas and consecutive hypoxia and hypercapnia arises after administration. An effective anxiolytic agent reduces the dose of anesthetic needed to induce general anesthesia, which

may otherwise lead to an increased likelihood of cardiovascular complications [9].

Tracheal extubation should be performed only when the patient is conscious, communicative, and breathing spontaneously with an adequate tidal volume and oxygenation [9,21]. Respiratory depression and repetitive apnea often occur directly after extubation in patients with OSA. Use of opiates increase this risk, and intravenous administration may cause delayed (4–12 hours after administration) respiratory depression [8,9,23]. It is believed that opiates should only be used when nonsteroidal anti-inflammatory drugs or regional anesthesia cannot be administrated. In some cases it may be wise to titrate short-acting opioid variants until pain sensation is sufficiently diminished. If nonsteroidal anti-inflammatory drugs can be used, this allows a reduction by 20% to 25% of opioids after major surgery [8]. Narcotic reversal agents should be used with caution. The duration of action may be less than longer-acting narcotic agents, and the patient may have a reduced sensorium and airway instability after the reversal has worn off [20].

Ostermeier and coworkers [8] state that patients with OSA are at an increased risk of developing respiratory problems postoperatively in the absence of pain. Pain prevents the rebound of REM sleep and diminishes stage 3 and 4 sleep, which also predisposes the collapse of the upper airway, around the third postoperative day. Use of nasal continuous positive airway pressure preoperatively and directly postoperatively reduces the risk of developing respiratory depression [28].

Respiratory depression with transient apnea occurs frequently in OSA patients and may be more

Table 4
Comparison of incidence of respiratory depression from IV PCA with basal (continuous) infusion and IV PCA without basal infusion

Study	Respiratory depression rates	
	IV PCA with basal infusion	IV PCA without basal infusion
Sidebotham, et al (1997) (respiratory depression <8 breaths/min)	3 (1.09%) of 276	11 (0.19%) of 5759 (Fischer's exact test, $P < .05$)
Schug and Torrie (1993) (respiratory depression requiring use of narcotic antagonist)	1.4% (approximately)	0.27% (Fischer's exact test, $P < .05$)
Fleming and Coombs (1992) (respiratory depression requiring use of narcotic antagonist; all patients had respiratory rate <6 breaths/min)	3 (3.8%) of 78	3 (0.29%) of 1044 (Fischer's exact test, $P < .01$)

Abbreviations: IV, intravenous; PCA, patient-controlled analgesia.
Data from Hagle ME, Lehr VT, Brubakken K, et al. Respiratory depression in adult patients with intravenous patient-controlled analgesia. Orthopaedic Nursing 2004;23:18–27.

likely with the use of opioids [8,31,32]. Ostermeier and coworkers [8] go on to state that during case review, respiratory depression occurred after a prolonged period of time up to 48 hours after the start of epidural administration of opioids and after earlier documentation of stable vital signs. Delayed respiratory depression has also been reported after intravenous administration of morphine. There are conflicting data regarding the use of epidural opioids in OSA patients. In the three case studies, Ostermeier and coworkers [8] showed that the patients did not demonstrate any of the usual signs of decreased ventilatory frequency, which normally leads to severe respiratory depression after epidural opioids.

In two reports when a basal infusion with intravenous patient-controlled analgesia was studied separately from intravenous patient-controlled analgesia without basal infusion, there was a lower rate of respiratory depression when intravenous patient-controlled analgesia was used without basal infusion (Table 4). Intravenous patient-controlled analgesia with a basal infusion significantly increases the risk of respiratory depression [24]. Meoli and coworkers [20] suggest that carefully establishing dosing limits related to airway and respiratory stability is essential if using patient-controlled analgesia.

Summary

OSA is a common problem affecting all ages, particularly in conjunction with other pre-existing conditions. The outcome of the syndrome may be severe. A further understanding of the morbidity and mortality associated with this OSA is important. Compounding the disorder with the added insult of surgery, anesthesia, analgesia, and sedation requires the medical team continuously to re-evaluate this particular patient population. The understanding of many commonly used pharmacology agents with this population is warranted. Prudent care is essential in the perioperative setting. Patients with OSA present a unique challenge for the medical team taking care of this patient population. Early recognition of risk factors for OSA, the reason for hospitalization, pharmacology, and understanding the pathogenesis of OSA can prevent major complications in this patient population. OSA can be first identified, aggravated, or intensified by the effects of sedation, analgesics, and anesthetic agents, which may lead to life-threatening cardiopulmonary complications. A team approach to caring for this population is essential. Communication among the various members of the health care team regarding findings and observation is necessary.

References

[1] Young T, Palta M, Dempsey J, et al. The occurrence of sleep-disordered breathing among middle-aged adults. N Engl J Med 1993;328:1230–5.

[2] Young T, Peppard P, Gottlieb D. Epidemiology of obstructive sleep apnea. Am J Respir Crit Care Med 2002;165:1217–39.

[3] Chokroverty S. An overview of sleep. In: Chokroverty S, editor. Sleep disorders medicine: basic science, technical considerations, and clinical aspects. 2nd edition. Boston: Butterworth-Heinemann; 1999. p. 7–20.

[4] Shneerson J. Handbook of sleep medicine. Cambridge: Blackwell; 2000.

[5] Robinson A, Guilleminaut C. Obstructive sleep apnea. In: Chokroverty S, editor. Sleep disorders medicine: basic science, technical considerations, and clinical aspects. 2nd edition. Boston: Butterworth-Heinemann; 1999. p. 331–53.

[6] Chokroverty S. Physiologic changes in sleep. In: Chokroverty S, editor. Sleep disorders medicine: basic science, technical considerations, and clinical aspects. 2nd edition. Boston: Butterworth-Heinemann; 1999. p. 95–125.

[7] Chokroverty S. Sleep, breathing and neurologic disorders. In: Chokroverty S, editor. Sleep disorders medicine: basic science, technical considerations, and clinical aspects. 2nd edition. Boston: Butterworth-Heinemann; 1999. p. 509–71.

[8] Ostermeier A, Roizen M, Hautkappe M, et al. Three sudden postoperative respiratory arrests associated with epidural opioid in patients with sleep apnea. Anesth Analg 1997;85:452–60.

[9] Herder C, Schmeck J, Appleboom D, et al. Risks of general anaesthesia in people with obstructive sleep apnea. BMJ 2004;329:955–9.

[10] Tanigawa T, Tachibana N, Yamagishi K, et al. Usual alcohol consumption and arterial desaturations during sleep. JAMA 2004;292:923–5.

[11] Miyata S, Noda A, Ito N, et al. REM sleep is impaired by a small amount of alcohol in young women sensitive to alcohol. Intern Med 2004;43:679–84.

[12] Taasan V, Block A, Boysen P, et al. Alcohol increases sleep apnea and oxygen desaturations in asymptomatic men. Am J Med 1981;71:240–5.

[13] Keenan S. Polysomnographic: technique: an overview. In: Chokroverty S, editor. Sleep disorders medicine: basic science, technical considerations, and clinical aspects. 2nd edition. Boston: Butterworth-Heinemann; 1999. p. 149–69.

[14] American Thoracic Society, Medical Section of the American Lung Association. Indications and standards for cardiopulmonary sleep studies. Am Rev Respir Dis 1989;139:559–68.

[15] Young T, Skatrud J, Peppard P. Risk factors for obstructive sleep apnea in adults. JAMA 2004;291:2013–6.

[16] Johns M. A new method for measuring daytime sleepiness: the Epworth sleepiness scale. Sleep 1991; 14:540–5.

[17] Exar EN, Collop NA. The upper airway resistance syndrome. Chest 1999;115:1127–39.

[18] Eastwood P, Szollosi I, Platt P, et al. Comparison of upper airway collapse during general anaesthesia and sleep. Lancet 2002;359:1207–9.

[19] Jain S, Dhand R. Perioperative treatment of patients with obstructive sleep apnea. Curr Opin Pulm Med 2004;10:482–8.

[20] Meoli A, Rosen C, Kristo D, et al. Upper airway management of the adult patient with obstructive sleep apnea in the perioperative period: avoiding complications. Sleep 2003;26:1060–5.

[21] Loadsman J, Hillman D. Anaesthesia and sleep apnoea. Br J Anaesth 2001;86:254–66.

[22] Greenblatt DJ, Harmatz JS, Shapiro L, et al. Sensitivity to triazolam in the elderly. N Engl J Med 1991;324: 1691–8.

[23] Charney D, Mihic S, Harris RA. Hypnotics and sedatives. In: Hardman J, Goodman-Gilman A, Limbird L, editors. Goodman & Gilman's the pharmacological basis of therapeutics. 10th edition. New York: McGraw-Hill; 2001. p. 402–5.

[24] Sanofi-Synthelabo. Bridgewater (NJ): Zolpidem package insert; 2002.

[25] Waters K, McBrien F, Stewart P, et al. Effects of OSA, inhalation anesthesia, and fentanyl on the airway and ventilation of children. J Appl Physiol 2002;92: 1987–94.

[26] Gupta RM, Parvizi J, Hanssen AD, et al. Postoperative complications in patients with obstructive sleep apnea syndrome undergoing hip or knee replacement: a case-control study. Mayo Clin Proc 2001;76:897–905.

[27] Knill R, Moote C, Skinner M, et al. Anesthesia with abdominal surgery leads to intense REM sleep during the first postoperative week. Anesthesiology 1990;73: 52–61.

[28] Rennotte M, Baele P, Aubert G, et al. Nasal continuous positive airway pressure in the perioperative management of patient with obstructive sleep apnea submitted to surgery. Chest 1995;107:367–74.

[29] Hiremath AS, Hillman DR, James AL, et al. Relationship between difficult tracheal intubation and obstructive sleep apnoea. Br J Anaesth 1998;80:606–11.

[30] Eastwood P, Szollosi I, Platt P, et al. Comparison of upper airway collapse during general anaesthesia and sleep. Lancet 2002;359:1207–9.

[31] Sharma V, Galli W, Haber A, et al. Unexpected risks during administration of conscious sedation: previously undiagnosed obstructive sleep apnea. Ann Intern Med 2003;139:707–8.

[32] VanDercar D, Martinez A, DeLisser E. Sleep apnea syndromes: a potential contradiction for patient controlled analgesia. Anesthesiology 1991;74:623–4.

ELSEVIER
SAUNDERS

Crit Care Nurs Clin N Am 17 (2005) 279–285

CRITICAL CARE
NURSING CLINICS
OF NORTH AMERICA

Sedation and Patient Safety

Debora Simmons, RN, MSN, CCRN, CCNS

*The Institute for Healthcare Excellence, The University of Texas MD Anderson Cancer Center, 1515 Holcombe, Unit 141,
Houston, TX 77030–4437, USA*

The Eindhoven classification system provides a basic framework for approaching safety within systems. The Eindhoven classification was originally developed for industrial applications and has been used extensively in the chemical industry and has been cited within Institute of Medicine reports [1]. A medical modified Eindhoven classification scale is used for the root causes identification in the Medical Event Reporting System for Transfusion Medicine transfusion event reporting system [2].Causal codes, such as used in the Eindhoven scale, are useful as a framework for gathering data, standardizing investigations, and collecting aggregates of data to examine clusters of events [3]. In addition, the simplicity of the Eindhoven codes allows for use of readily available information for nurses and facilitates the analysis.

According to the Eindhoven scale, root causes are classified into three major categories or domains: (1) technical (equipment, software, forms); (2) organizational (policies, procedures, and protocols); and (3) human causes (knowledge-based, rule-based, and skill-based). The three domains are useful in classifying contributing factors and organizing causes. Because the initial reaction in an error event is to focus on the human factors, it is important to consider the first two domains before looking at human factor contributions (Table 1).

Technical risks to safety

The Eindhoven classification considers technical failures as being related to the "hardware" of care

including mechanical devices, forms, and software. Medical devices are a major safety concern both in consideration of a primary failure of the device and as a failure in human-machine interactions.

The Food and Drug Administration (FDA) maintains surveillance over medical devices and receives over 80,000 reports annually regarding failures, serious injuries, and deaths related to medical devices [4]. The Institute of Medicine in Canada reviewed 425 incident reports of parental, epidural, insulin, and patient-controlled analgesia pumps and found 23 deaths and 135 injuries related to technical features of pumps [5]. Both groups found similar problems related to devices. The FDA MedWatch program collects suspicious and confirmed device-related problems and provides a free public service news alert [6]. There must be caution in reviewing device failures in that reports of device failures are not necessarily the readily apparent cause [7]. A careful investigation into causes is always suggested, and to do so, a complete review of factors is necessary.

Despite increasingly strenuous testing and device design requirements, failures related to human interaction with devices continue. Broad categories of failures include factors related to devices, external factors, support system failures, user errors, and tampering or sabotage [7]. Commonly cited failures include

1. Lack of standardized devices in a facility (eg, the on switch on one device may be the off switch on a similar device of a different model or manufacturer) [4]
2. Lack of safe default settings so alarms that are suspended may not return to audible levels (software default settings) [4,8]
3. Designs that allow for free flow of medications [5,8]

No funding support was received for this paper.
E-mail address: dsimmon@mdanderson.org

4. Use of multiple infusion devices with similar numerical displays and poor labeling (labeling not easily read while the device is in use) [5].
5. Tubing that is similar to different infusion devices (epidural, arterial, and intravenous) [5].

Patient-controlled analgesia (PCA) has applicability and efficacy and is used in many settings in acute care. Unfortunately, PCA pump errors are often severe and can be fatal. Human factors analysis of pump failures reported to the FDA as reported by Brown and coworkers [9] included failures in programming and setup. In sentinel events related to programming of PCA pumps resulting in overdoses of narcotics, human factor design was found at the root of programming error [10].

The United States Pharmacopoeia examined medication errors submitted to its MEDMARX and United States Pharmacopoeia Medication Errors Reporting Program and identified the most common types of errors with PCA devices as improper dose or quantity (38.9%); unauthorized drug (18.4%); and omission error (17.6%). Included in the case reports were instances of wrong drug identification, programming errors, and inappropriate use of the demand feature.

PCA by proxy is the practice of using the demand feature for the patient. Several case studies are found in the literature that include family members and nursing staff administering doses without the request of the patient [11]. The intent of PCA is to have the patient be able to control a preset administration. To prevent intentional or unintentional tampering, locking keypads and mechanisms to prevent changing settings are recommended by the FDA. Errors have been made with inexperienced or untrained staff not being able to lock these features, and staff that did not understand the use of the PCA [12]. Although designed for safe use by patients, there are cases in which administration is initiated by nursing staff, which negates the fail-safe measure of a patient not using the demand feature because they become sedated.

Box 1. Common PCA-related safety issues

PCA by proxy
Improper patient selection
Inadequate monitoring
Inadequate patient education
Drug product mix-ups
Practice-related problems
Device design flaws
Inadequate staff training
Prescription errors

The FDA and Institute for Safe Medication Practices report a case of a 72-year-old woman who received morphine through PCA after surgery, and died of an overdose after nurses pushed the PCA button and delivered frequent doses of morphine for 48 hours. The patient suffered an arrest and seizure and died several months later [13]. The Joint Commission on Accreditation of Healthcare Organizations (JCAHO) recently issued a sentinel event alert regarding PCA by proxy and reported 6069 PCA errors reported to the United States Pharmacopoeia with 460 resulting fatalities (Box 1) [14].

Although identified early in the Institute of Medicine reports, device-human interactive failures continue frequently in health care [4]. Risk of both errors can be mitigated by human factors specific design and failure mode and effects analysis (Table 2).

Organizational factors

Organizational practices are often described as latent factors in errors. Latent factors are decisions,

Table 1
Major categories

Eindhoven classification basic categories		Code
Technical	Equipment, software, forms	T
Organizational	Policies, procedures, and protocols	O
Human causes	Knowledge-based, rule-based, and skill-based	H

Table 2
Eindhoven technical factors

Technical subcategories	Description refers to physical items, such as equipment, physical installations, software, materials, labels, and forms	Code
External	Technical failures beyond the control and responsibility of the investigating organization	TEX
Design	Failures caused by poor design of equipment, software, labels, or forms	TD
Construction	Correct design was not followed accurately during construction	TC
Materials	Material defects not classified under TD or TC	TM

policies, and procedures that lie dormant within an organization and only become apparent when an error occurs [15]. Latent factors are missed if investigations are not performed with a methodology for discovery. Latent and organizational factors are also important for proactive interventions because they are controllable factors.

Organizational failures contributing to risk have been cited in Institute of Medicine literature and culture research [4]. "Keeping Patients Safe: Transforming the Work Environment of Nurses," recently published by the Institute of Medicine, recognizes lack of surveillance of patients as a major contributor to safety [16]. Surveillance of patients is highly influenced by organizational culture, policies, procedures, and practices for staffing, training, documentation, and workload [16]. The failure to monitor patients is termed "failure to rescue." As workload increases with acuity, tasks, or numbers of patients, the ability of nursing staff to recognize changes in conditions and respond to changing conditions decreases. Aiken and coworkers [17] concluded in the study of acute hospitals with high patient-to-nurse ratios that surgical patients experience higher risk-adjusted 30-day mortality and failure-to-rescue rates. Failure to rescue has further been explored by Needleman and coworkers [18] and validated as an indicator of quality in acute care surgical patients by Silber.

Policies and procedures that do not support the work of care by setting untenable standards are a threat to safe care. In the case of sedation and analgesia administration, care should be given to avoid creating policies that are not meaningful or able to be followed within the context of the work environment. "Work-a-rounds" are created by staff to complete tasks when they are not able to complete the work as required by policy or time limitations. When work-a-rounds become common practice there are critical safety means that are left out of the work flow, creating hazardous conditions.

Medication errors

Medication errors are categorized within four action phases: (1) prescribing, (2) transcribing, (3) dispensing, and (4) administration. Errors are found within all phases of the medication process; however, the detection of an error may occur more frequently at the point of administration. Organizational factors influence each stage of the administration process from prescribing, transcription, dispensing, and administration.

Prescribing errors related to analgesia and sedation include dosing errors, prescribing medications to which the patient is allergic, and prescribing inappropriate dosage forms. In a review of 11,186 confirmed medication-prescribing errors, narcotics were among the most common medication classes involved in errors [19]. Legibility, lack of information that is patient-specific or drug-specific, abbreviations, and order forms continue to be problematic [20].

Transcription errors include errors made by humans in transferring medications to pharmacy or to administration records. The Eindhoven classification categorizes errors in transfer of information as an organizational failure if the transfer is to new or inexperienced staff. Organizational practices that do not support adequate time or emphasis on information transfer can be a factor in failure to communicate.

Dispensing and administration errors include dispensing the wrong drug, substituting drugs with similar names, and providing differing concentrations of drugs. The JCAHO identifies latent factors related to safety with analgesia and sedation in the National Patient Safety Goals. Practices to increase safety related to sedation and anesthesia include

1. Standardizing and limiting the number of drug concentrations available in the organization.
2. Identifying and annually reviewing a list of look-alike–sound-alike drugs used in the organization, and taking action to prevent errors involving the interchange of these drugs.
3. Prohibiting abbreviations that can be confusing and using a list of commonly understood abbreviations.

Cases of inadvertent administration of sufentanil instead of fentanyl during patient sedation or analgesia is prevalent in the literature [21]. Hydromorphone and morphine have been confused in a similar manner causing an overdose [20]. These include similarities in product packaging appearance and names of these two medications. Medication sound-alikes and look-alikes continue to be a source of potential error [21]. Drug formularies should be vigilantly monitored for look-alike and sound-alike medications until the pharmaceutical industry responds to this problem (Table 3).

Human factors

Human factors are often termed "active" because they happen in real time often without warning. An individual who performs perfectly at other times reliably makes an error eventually. For these reasons, the human interactions in errors are more

Table 3
Eindhoven classification of organizational errors

Eindhoven classification organizational factors	Description	Code
External	Failures at an organizational level beyond the control and responsibility of the investigating organization	OEX
Transfer of knowledge	Failures resulting from inadequate measures taken to ensure that situational or domain-specific knowledge or information is transferred to all new or inexperienced staff	OK
Protocols or procedures	Failures related to the quality and availability of the protocols within the department (too complicated, inaccurate, unrealistic, absent, or poorly presented)	OP
Management priorities	Internal management decisions in which safety is regulated in an inferior position in the face of conflicting demands or objectives; this conflicts between production needs and safety (eg, decisions about staffing levels)	OM
Culture	Failures resulting from collective approach to risk and attendant modes of behavior in the investigating organization	OC

difficult to understand and require patient investigation to uncover.

The Eindhoven classification system identifies a small spectrum of the range of human errors and this has been a criticism of its use in health care. In addition, it takes training and education in human factors to understand this classification. The need for this training has been newly realized by hospitals.

Knowledge-based errors

Errors in knowledge are cited in sedation and analgesia errors. When nurses use the PCA and de-mand for the patient, resulting in oversedation, this can be attributed to knowledge error on the part of the practitioner. Family members who administer PCA may also have knowledge deficits. Patients returning from procedures may not understand or remember PCA instructions.

Staff unfamiliar with oxygen saturation and implications for sedation are at risk for misinterpretation of readings. In addition, pulse oximetry is limited in its assessment values in patients with poor peripheral circulation. Decline in oxygen saturation may not be recognized as an indicator or may be disallowed as a factual reading. The increased technology assistance

Table 4
Eindhoven classification of human factors

Eindhoven classification human (active errors)	Description: errors or failures resulting from human behavior	Code
External	Human failures originating beyond the control and responsibility of the investigating organization	HEX
Knowledge-based behaviors, knowledge-based errors	The inability of an individual to apply existing knowledge to a novel situation	HKK
Rule-based behaviors	Incorrect fit between the individual's qualification, training, or education and a particular task	HRQ
Coordination	Lack of task coordination within a health care team within an organization	HRQ
Verification	Failures in the correct and complete assessment of a situation, including relevant conditions of the patient and materials to be sued before starting the intervention	HRV
Intervention	Failures that result from faulty tasks planning (selecting the wrong protocol) or execution (selecting the right protocol but carrying it out incorrectly)	
Monitoring	Failures during monitoring of the process or patient status during or after an intervention	HRM
Skill-based behaviors	Failures in performance of fine motor skills	HSS
Slips and trips	Failures in whole body movement	HSS HST
Patient-related factors	Failures related to patient characteristics or conditions that influence the treatment and are beyond the control of staff	PRF
Unclassifiable	Failures that cannot be classified in any other category	X

in patient monitoring cannot overcome the burden of clinical decisions based on those measures.

Patient-related factors

Pediatric patients fall victim to errors frequently because of decimal points being placed in the wrong position resulting in 10-fold overdoses [20]. In addition, rapid changes in body weight make calculations and the risk of error more frequent [20]. Drugs with long half-lives have been associated with pediatric deaths [22]. Adverse sedation events were frequently associated with drug overdoses and drug interactions, particularly when three or more drugs

Table 5
The Eindhoven classification model for a medical domain

Category	Description	Code
Latent errors	Errors that result from underlying system failures	
Technical	Refers to physical items, such as equipment, physical installations, software, materials, labels, and forms	
External	Technical failures beyond the control and responsibility of the investigating organization	TEX
Design	Failures caused by poor design of equipment, software, labels, or forms	TD
Construction	Construction failures despite correct design	TC
Materials	Material defects not classified under TD or TC	TM
Organizational		
External	Failures at an organizational level beyond the control and responsibility of the investigating organization	OEX
Transfer of knowledge	Failures resulting from inadequate measures taken to ensure that situational or domain-specific knowledge or information is transferred to all new or inexperienced staff	OK
Protocols and procedures	Failures related to the quality and availability of the protocols within the department (too complicated, inaccurate, unrealistic, absent, or poorly presented)	OP
Management priorities	Internal management decisions in which safety is relegated to an inferior position in the face of conflicting demands or objectives; this is a conflict between production needs and safety (eg, decisions about staffing levels)	OM
Culture	Failures resulting from the collective approach to risk and attendant modes of behavior in the investigating organization	OC
Active errors (human)	Errors or failures resulting from human behavior	
External	Human failures originating beyond the control and responsibility of the investigating organization	HEX
Knowledge-based behaviors		
Knowledge-based errors	The inability of an individual to apply existing knowledge to a novel situation	HKK
Rule-based behaviors		
Qualification	Incorrect fit between an individual's qualifications, training, or education and a particular task	HRQ
Coordination	Lack of task coordination within a health care team in an organization	HRC
Verification	Failures in the correct and complete assessment of a situation, including relevant conditions of the patient and materials to be used, before starting the intervention	HRV
Intervention	Failures that result from faulty task planning (selecting the wrong protocol) or execution (selecting the right protocol but carrying it out incorrectly)	HRI
Monitoring	Failures during monitoring of the process or patient status during or after the intervention	HRM
Skill-based behaviors		
Slips	Failures in performance of fine motor skills	HSS
Tripping	Failures in whole-body movements	HST
Other		
Patient-related factor	Failures related to patient characteristics or conditions that influence treatment and are beyond the control of staff	PRF
Unclassifiable	Failures that cannot be classified in any other category	X

were used in a study of 118 case reports from the adverse drug reporting system of the United States Pharmacopoeia [22]. Recommendations from this study group include uniform monitoring and training standards regardless of the area of patient care, standards of care, scope of practice, resource management, or reimbursement for sedation and should be based on the depth of sedation achieved (ie, the degree of vigilance and resuscitation skills required) rather than on the drug class, route of drug administration, practitioner, or venue [22].

The elderly are known to have vulnerability related to polypharmacy that increases the risk in interactions, pathophysiologic changes in body mass, and chemistry [23]. Analgesics and drugs that affect central nervous system function are often overprescribed [24]. Benzodiazepines are among the more commonly prescribed drugs for the elderly despite the risk of respiratory depression (Table 4) [23].

Approaching safety in sedation

Classification systems provide a framework for considering aspects of safety and a path for investigating issues. Investigation can be guided by the classification system to prevent short sightedness and to overlook important issues. Examining interventions for safety in delivery of sedation and analgesia can be accomplished using the Eindhoven classification to guide results. Classification systems define the domains of investigation [3].

Proactive approaches to safety include using Failure Mode and Effects Analysis to define, assess, and rate failure points. The steps of Failure Mode and Effects Analysis include a definition of the problem, process, or new element, such as a new pump. The Eindhoven classification can be used to frame findings during the exercise and present them for criticality scoring.

Reactive assessment of errors benefits from a defined classification system. Using the three domains as a base for investigation creates a structured methodology for root cause analysis and prevents omitting one domain. It is human nature to begin with the question of "whom"? The Eindhoven framework begins with technical factors moving to organizational and then human factors. Disciplined use of this path prevents focus on the human domain.

Prioritization of interventions also benefits from classification. A common formula for prioritizing risk is frequency multiplied by severity. As a reactive or proactive process ensues, using the Eindhoven

classification forms a base for aggregating results in each domain.

Summary

Increasingly, information is provided by specialized reports and internal investigations that apply to mission-critical safety issues; the enormous challenge is dissemination of information to facilitate application at the point of care. Providers now have an extensive data gathering process whether it is proactive or reactive. Using Eindhoven classification schema to aggregate the results of these efforts or aggregate the alerts from sources is a method for investigating safety concerns and errors and aggregating data for risk assessment and prioritization (Table 5).

References

[1] Aspden P, Corrigan J, Wolcott J, et al. Patient safety: achieving a new standard of care. Washington (DC): National Academies Press; 2003.

[2] MERS-TM. Root causes EMC Table. In: MERS-TM; 2004.

[3] Kaplan HS, Rabin Fastman B. Organization of event reporting data for sense making and system improvement. Qual Saf Health Care 2003;12:68–72.

[4] Kohn L, Corrigan J, Donaldson M, editors. To err is human: building a safer health system. Washington (DC): National Academy Press; 2000.

[5] Canada I. High alert drugs and infusion pumps. In: Canada I, editor. Institute for Safe Medication Practices; 2004.

[6] Food and Drug Administration. MedWatch. Washington: US Food and Drug Administration; 2005.

[7] Goodman G. Medical device error. Crit Care Clin 2002;14:407–16.

[8] JCAHO. 2004 National patient safety goals. Oakbrook Terrace (IL): The Joint Commission on Accreditation of Healthcare Organizations; 2004.

[9] Brown SLB, Parmentier M, Taylor CJ. Human error and patient-controlled analgesia pumps. Journal of Infusion Nursing 1997;20:311–6.

[10] Vincente KJ, Kada-Bekhaled K, Hillel G, et al. Programming errors contribute to death from patient-controlled analgesia: case report and estimate of probability. Can J Anaesth 2003;50:328–32.

[11] Institute for Safe Medication Practices. More on avoiding opiate toxicity with PCA by proxy. Huntingdon Valley (PA): ISMP; 2004.

[12] Food and Drug Administration. Safety tip: patient-controlled analgesia (PCA) pumps with keypad locking mechanisms. Washington: US Food and Drug Administration; 2003.

[13] Food and Drug Administration. Hazards in patient-controlled analgesia. Washington: US Food and Drug Administration; 2002.

[14] JCAHO. Sentinel event alert: patient controlled analgesia by proxy. Washington (DC): JCAHO; 2004.

[15] Reason J. Human error: models and management. BMJ 2000;320:768–70.

[16] Institute of Medicine. Keeping patients safe: transforming the work environment of nurses. Washington (DC): National Academies Press; 2004.

[17] Aiken LHCS, Sloane DM, Sochalski J, et al. Hospital nurse staffing and patient mortality, nurse burnout, and job dissatisfaction. JAMA 2002;288:1987–93.

[18] Needleman J, Buerhaus P, Mattke S, et al. Nurse-staffing levels and the quality of care in hospitals. N Engl J Med 2002;346:1715–22.

[19] Lesar TS, Lomaestro BM, Pohl H. Medication-prescribing errors in a teaching hospital: a 9-year experience. Arch Intern Med 1997;157:1569–76.

[20] Cohen M. Medication errors. 1st edition. Washington: American Pharmaceutical Foundation; 1999.

[21] Chisholm CD, Klanduch F. Inadvertent administration of sufentanil instead of fentanyl during sedation/analgesia in a community hospital emergency department: a report of two cases. Acad Emerg Med 2000; 7:1282–4.

[22] Cote CJ, Karl HW, Notterman DA, et al. Adverse sedation events in pediatrics: analysis of medications used for sedation. Pediatrics 2000;106:633–44.

[23] Hall C. Special considerations for the geriatric population. Crit Care Nurs Clin North Am 2002;14:427–34.

[24] Goulding MR. Inappropriate medication prescribing for elderly ambulatory care patients. Arch Intern Med 2004;164:306–12.

**ELSEVIER
SAUNDERS**

Crit Care Nurs Clin N Am 17 (2005) 287–296

**CRITICAL CARE
NURSING CLINICS**
OF NORTH AMERICA

Complications of Sedation and Critical Illness

Jan Foster, PhD, RN, CNS, CCRN, CCN[a,b,*]

[a]*College of Nursing, Texas Woman's University, 1130 John Freeman Boulevard, Houston, TX 77030, USA*
[b]*Nursing Inquiry and Intervention, 58 Aberdeen Crossing, The Woodlands, TX 77381, USA*

Dave, a 41-year-old otherwise healthy man, presented to the emergency department of a small community hospital with shortness of breath and altered mental status. He was placed on a non-rebreather oxygen mask, but because he could not maintain his oxygen saturation, he was intubated and supported with mechanical ventilation on maximum settings. He was diagnosed with pneumonia and sepsis, and over the next several weeks developed acute respiratory distress syndrome, empyema, and sinusitis. Management was complicated by allergy to appropriate antibiotics, along with nicotine and presumed opiate or benzodiazepine withdrawal, which Dave took for chronic cervical neck and back pain resulting from a previous injury. He was extremely febrile and tachycardic for days, necessitating heavy doses of lorazepam, propofol, and occasional doses of cisatracurium or pancuronium to facilitate the work of breathing. Three weeks later Dave was weaned from sedation and extubated. This was not, however, the end of his medical problems.

Dave experienced extreme muscle wasting, leaving him very weak and unstable during ambulation attempts. He reported disturbed sleep patterns with frequent bizarre dreams throughout and following sedation administration, leaving him so fatigued it interfered with rehabilitation during the day. Focal weakness in his right leg became apparent, along with foot drop. Through electromyography and nerve conduction studies it was determined he had peroneal nerve injury. Physical therapy was initiated in the acute care hospital setting and continued in a rehabilitation facility following discharge. Eight years later, impaired dorsiflexion interferes with safe operation of a motor vehicle.

Although use of sedation is a necessary component of care for the critically ill, careful and vigilant monitoring to guard against oversedation is necessary to prevent complications not only in the immediate acute care setting, but also to minimize long-term problems, delay return to functional status, and jeopardize quality of life following critical illness. Despite prudent use of sedatives and neuromuscular blocking agents, with dosing guided by a subjective sedation scale and peripheral nerve monitoring, respectively, parenteral and enteral nutrition, and physical therapy, Dave suffered common long-term sequelae of critical illness, heavy sedation, and neuromuscular blockade.

Oversedation

Oversedation complicates the clinical course for patients during the critical period of illness and may contribute to long-term problems. Risks of oversedation for critically ill patients include hypotension, bradycardia, coma, respiratory depression, ileus, renal failure, venous stasis, and immune suppression [1]. Psychologic complications associated with excessive sedation include tolerance and tachyphylaxis; withdrawal syndrome; and rarely, paradoxical and psychotic reactions [1,2].

Prolonged sedation may occur after cessation of some medications even when carefully titrated. For example, prolonged effects have been reported with the use of midazolam, caused by altered pharmaco-

* College of Nursing, Texas Woman's University, 1130 John Freeman Boulevard, Houston, TX 77030.
E-mail address: jfoster@twu.edu

kinetics in critically ill patients or accumulation of active metabolites [1]. Decreased organ perfusion and organ dysfunction, particularly hepatic and renal, contribute to accumulation of drugs and their active metabolites, which prolongs the sedation effects after terminating the drugs. Concurrent administration of certain medications commonly used in critical care, such as cimetidine and erythromycin, prolongs the sedative effects of midazolam [1].

Respiratory complications include reduced response to carbon dioxide levels, decreased minute ventilation, and apnea, which generally are not problematic in the ICU because patients are closely monitored or are supported with mechanical ventilation. In ventilated patients with respiratory depression caused by oversedation, however, weaning can be delayed. In a comparison of midazolam with propofol, Barrientos-Vega and colleagues [3] found prolonged weaning times for both groups, even with titrating level of sedation to a Ramsay Score of 4 or 5 (asleep and responsive to voice or pain). Weaning time for patients following propofol infusion (N = 25), measured from discontinuation of the drug to extubation, was 34.8 ± 29.4 hours. For patients in the midazolam group the weaning time was significantly longer (97.9 ± 54.6 hours [$P = .0001$]).

Neuromuscular impairment

Critically ill individuals have multiple reasons for the development of skeletal muscle weakness, stemming from both neurophysiologic and myopathic abnormalities. The causes are multifactorial and include inactivity, local and systemic inflammatory mediator release during sepsis and other severe insult, multiorgan dysfunction, steroid use, neuromuscular blockade, and a combination of factors [4–8].

Critical illness polyneuropathy has been described in the literature for at least two decades. It is characterized by severe weakness in both proximal and distal muscles of the extremities, deep tendon areflexia, and normal sensory nerve conduction, along with intact cranial nerve, cerebellar, brainstem, and cerebral hemisphere function. Weak diaphragmatic muscles interfere with ventilator weaning [9]. Electromyography shows evidence of diffuse axonal degeneration of peripheral nerves. In a recent study of long-term survivors of prolonged critical illness, Fletcher and associates [10] found motor or sensory deficits in 59% of 22 patients studied. Twenty-two had electromyographic indications of chronic partial denervation associated with axonal neuropathy. They concluded that critical illness polyneuropathy causing

extreme weakness can last for as long as 5 years after critical illness.

In addition to critical illness polyneuropathy, critical illness myopathy accounts for severe weakness associated with critical illness. It too is linked with sepsis and multiorgan dysfunction, along with steroid use, which have muscle-necrotizing properties [11]. Critical illness myopathy is suspected by clinical presentation of extreme muscle weakness and conclusively determined by direct muscle stimulation during electrophysiology studies and muscle biopsy. Electrodiagnostic findings include decreased muscle membrane excitability, and biopsy results reveal myofilament loss [12,13]. In a retrospective study of all documented cases of critical illness neuromyopathy in one facility (N = 30) over a 5-year period, the investigators found 8 cases of critical illness polyneuropathy, 15 cases of critical illness myopathy, and 7 cases of mixed critical illness polyneuropathy and critical illness myopathy [14]. Similarly, other researchers found in a review of 46 postcritically ill patients that 26 could be classified into three groups. Twelve subjects had evidence of purely critical illness myopathy, 1 critical illness polyneuropathy, and 13 subjects with combined critical illness myopathy and critical illness polyneuropathy [12].

These studies indicate that critically ill patients are at risk for severe neuromuscular impairment caused by complex processes that have not yet been thoroughly explained. Furthermore, severe weakness frequently goes undiagnosed because of the presence of many confounding clinical issues and priorities, such as concern for hemodynamic stability and oxygenation and ventilation. Oversedation masks the presentation of severe weakness, delays diagnosis and management, and contributes to a cycle of inactivity.

Disuse muscle atrophy

Prolonged bed rest and immobility associated with sedative use in critically ill patients induces severe muscle inactivity, followed by disuse atrophy, and further impairment of physical mobility [15]. Skeletal muscle adapts to changes in activity with structural alterations, which in turn effects mechanical properties and influences local muscle properties and metabolic processes. In addition, prolonged bed rest triggers systemic physiologic consequences, which complicate fluid and electrolyte balance, hemodynamic stability, and ventilation and oxygenation [16]. Additionally, patients are at increased risk for venous stasis and thromboembolic events, skin breakdown, and atelectasis.

Two components of decreased muscle activity include hypodynamia (a decrease in weight bearing) and hypokinesia (a decrease in movement and range of motion) [15]. When there is a reduction in movement or weight bearing, skeletal muscle undergoes plastic changes (remodeling that corresponds to functional changes) by reducing its mass through increased protein degradation coupled with decreased protein synthesis [17]. Disuse atrophy results in loss of muscle mass caused by a reduction in muscle cell diameter and the number of fibers. Shrinking muscle mass begins quickly after activity change, within the first 4 hours, and is most severe during the third to seventh day of inactivity [18,19].

Bedridden critically ill patients are subject to both hypodynamic and hypokinetic muscle inactivity leading to disuse atrophy. Both are compounded by the use of sedatives, which is further aggravated by an extended weaning process. Assessment for disuse atrophy is accomplished at the bedside through traditional muscle strength evaluation. Biochemical markers for evaluation of muscle damage include creatine kinase and troponin levels. Quantification of muscle damage may be done through computerized dynamometry, and nuclear MRI provides examination of muscle tissue [18].

Severe muscle weakness stemming from critical illness develops from multiple factors. Identification may be shrouded by patient variables, such as sedatives, neuromuscular blockade, and manifestations of critical illness or injury. Severe muscle weakness may go unnoticed because of clinician lack of awareness of the problem and focus on other clinical priorities. Intervention for muscle atrophy in the acute and critical period of illness is a challenge, even with identification of the problem, because strenuous exercise of atrophied muscle may induce muscle fiber damage [18]. Patients with severe muscle weakness require long-term physical therapy for restoration of balance, strengthening and conditioning, and return to baseline function.

Cost factors

When evaluating costs of sedation in the ICU, both shelf costs of the drugs and costs related to care must be taken into consideration. Prolonged recovery time from sedatives may necessitate longer duration of ventilator support, ICU length of stay, and hospital length of stay, escalating the costs of treatment. Accurately accounting for drug-associated costs is a

challenge; considerations include supplies, such as bags, syringes, tubing; equipment, such as pumps and monitors; and personnel labor costs of medication ordering, mixing, and dispensing, syringe handling, manipulation of administration sets, site assessment and care, trips to the patient bedside, and so forth. In attempts to capture and compare costs of sedatives, often many of these factors are overlooked. For example, in a study reported by Cernaianu and coworkers [20], even though lorazepam ($1.85 per milligram) cost more than midazolam ($1.73 per milligram), smaller doses of lorazepam were needed to achieve effective sedation. The authors concluded that intermittent injection of lorazepam was more cost effective. They did not take into account, however, the supply, equipment, and personnel costs of the drugs. In another report, the amount of time patients were oversedated (Ramsay Score 5–6) was less in patients who received midazolam than patients receiving lorazepam (18% versus 36%, $P = .009$) [21]. When recovery costs are taken into account, this study suggests midazolam is a more cost-effective choice of sedation.

Preventing complications of sedation

Appropriate sedation is a multidimensional problem; clinicians and researchers must look for solutions in a variety of places. Assessment of sedation with a combination of instruments, selecting the appropriate medication and method of delivery, and an individualized plan are tools currently available to best meet patient's needs. More work is needed, however, in each of these areas.

Measuring sedation

Appropriate sedation begins with assessment for underlying causes of agitation, such as pain, anxiety, hypoxemia, fever, and withdrawal syndromes. Next, caregivers must communicate the goals of sedation. The critical care team must agree on the end points of adequate sedation and use the same measures of assessment. Over 30 subjective scales for measurement of sedation level have been described in the medical literature [22]. Formal evaluation for both reliability and validity is reported, however, in only eight instruments: the Ramsay [23], Harris [24], Sedation-Agitation [25], Motor Activity Assessment [26], Vancouver Interaction and Calmness [27], COMFORT [28], Richmond Agitation Scale (RASS) [29], and ATICE [30]. Some, however, hold more reliability and validity than others.

Table 1
Ramsay sedation scale

Level	Response
1	Awake and anxious, agitated, or restless
2	Awake, cooperative, accepting ventilation, oriented, and tranquil
3	Awake; responds only to commands
4	Asleep; brisk response to light glabellar tap or loud auditory noise
5	Asleep; sluggish response to light glabellar tap or loud auditory stimulus but does not respond to painful stimulus
6	Asleep; no response to light glabellar tap or loud auditory stimulus

From Ramsay M, Savege T, Simpson BRJ, et al. Controlled sedation with alphaxalone/alphadolone. BMJ 1974;2: 656–9; with permission.

The Ramsay Sedation Scale is one of the earliest published tools for use in critically ill patients [23] and has undergone modification since initial publication. It is a six-scale tool with levels ranging from overt agitation to unresponsive coma (Table 1). The tool has been criticized because the levels are not mutually exclusive. For example, mild anxiety and extreme agitation fall into the same category (Ramsay 1), with the next level representative of desired goals of therapeutic sedation (Ramsay 2). Also, a patient can respond to commands (Ramsay 3), which may be a better indicator of cognition versus sedation, and at the same time be both anxious and restless (Ramsay 1), or asleep and responsive to glabellar tap (Ramsay 4).

The Harris scale was developed specifically for patients receiving mechanical ventilation and addresses three components of patient assessment: (1) general condition, (2) compliance with mechanical ventilation, and (3) response to endotracheal suctioning [24]. The general condition has six levels ranging from uncontrollable agitation to unarousable sedation (Box 1). The mechanical ventilation and endotracheal suction components each have four levels of sedation. The instrument has demonstrated strong interrater reliability on all three aspects of the scale: kappa = .90, $P < .001$ for sedation; and .91 and .83 ($P < .001$) for the mechanical ventilation and endotracheal suction segments of the scale. The sedation subscale has also shown strong agreement with two other scales: the Ramsay Scale ($r^2 = .83$, $P < .001$) and the Riker Sedation-Agitation Scale ($r^2 = .86$, $P < .001$).

The Riker Sedation-Agitation-Scale is a seven-point scale ranging from unarousable to dangerous sedation (Table 2) [31]. Strong points include its

mutually exclusive categories, behavioral examples provided as criteria for each score, and a symmetric range of sedation and agitation with a midpoint score of four for the patient who is "calm and cooperative" with degrees of agitation scored 5 through 7 and degrees of sedation scored 3 through 1, making the tool intuitively useful. The instrument shows sound interrater reliability (kappa = .92, $P < .001$) and correlates well with the Ramsay ($r^2 = .83$, $P < .001$) and Harris scales ($r^2 = .86$, $P < .001$).

The Motor Activity Assessment Scale (Table 3) is similar to the Riker Sedation-Agitation-Scale in that it measures sedation and agitation with a symmetric seven-level scale; the scores range from 0 to 6 instead of 1 to 7 [26]. It also provides

---

Box 1. Harris scale

General condition

1. Confused and uncontrollable
2. Anxious and agitated
3. Conscious, oriented, and calm
4. Asleep but arousable to speech, obeys commands
5. Asleep but responds to loud auditory stimulus or sternal pressure
6. Unarousable

Compliance with mechanical ventilation

1. Unable to control ventilation
2. Distressed, fighting ventilator
3. Coughing when moved but tolerating ventilation for most of the time
4. Tolerating movement

Response to endotracheal suctioning

1. Agitation, distress, prolonged coughing
2. Coughs, distressed, rapid recovery
3. Coughs, not distressed
4. No cough

From Harris E, O'Donnell C, Macmillan RR, et al. Use of propofol infusion for sedation of patients undergoing haemofiltration – Assessment of the effect of haemofiltration on the level of sedation on blood propofol concentration. J Drug Dev 1991;4(Suppl 3):37–9.

Table 2
Riker Sedation-Agitation-Scale

Level	Behaviors
7 Dangerous agitation	Pulls at endotracheal tube, tries to remove catheters, climbs over bed rail, strikes at staff, thrashes side-to-side
6 Very agitated	Does not calm, despite frequent verbal reminding of limits; requires verbal reminding of limits; requires physical restraints; bites endotracheal tube
5 Agitated	Anxious or mildly agitated, attempts to sit up, calms down to verbal instructions
4 Calm and cooperative	Calm, awakens easily, follows commands
3 Sedated	Difficult to arouse, awakens to verbal stimuli or gentle shaking but drifts off again, follows simple commands
2 Very sedated	Arouses to physical stimuli but does not communicate or follow commands, may move spontaneously
1 Unarousable	Minimal or no response to noxious stimuli, does not communicate or follow commands

From Fraser GL, Riker R. Monitoring sedation, agitation, analgesia, and delirium in critically ill adult patients. Crit Care Clin 2001;17:1−21.

behavioral descriptors for each score. Reliability of the Motor Activity Assessment Scale shows strong agreement among raters (kappa = .83, confidence interval 0.72 and 0.94) [26].

The Vancouver Interaction and Calmness Scale was developed in four phases, the final phase culminating in a symmetric scale of patient behaviors using a Likert scale for assessment of sedation [27]. With 302 observations on 34 mechanically ventilated adult patients in the ICU and subacute care unit, strong interrater reliability was established with an intraclass correlation coefficient of 0.90 and internal consistency of 0.95 (Table 4).

The COMFORT scale was developed in 1992 exclusively for pediatric patients and includes eight components of behaviors and physiologic parameters rated on a scale of 1 to 5 and includes alertness, calmness and agitation, movement, muscle tone, respiratory status, facial tension, blood pressure, and heart rate [28]. During testing of the instrument, strong reliability ($r = 0.84$, $P < .01$) and validity ($r = 0.75$, $P < .01$ when compared with a visual analog scale) were demonstrated [28].

A more recently developed scale, the RASS (Table 5), shows promising reliability and variable validity scores. The scale measures 10 items with levels ranging from combative to unarousable The instrument was initially evaluated in 192 patient

observations in medical, surgical, cardiac surgical, coronary, and neuroscience ICUs. Interrater reliability was high among five observers ($r = 0.922 - 0.983$, kappa=$0.64 - 0.82$) and validity was established through strong correlation with a visual analog scale illustrating levels of combativeness and unresponsiveness ($r = 0.84 - 0.98$) during the evaluation [29].

A scale to measure adaptation to the intensive care environment (ATICE) has demonstrated reliability, validity, and responsiveness to patient behavior. The instrument enhances bedside clinical assessment of tolerance to environmental stimuli and assists with sedation titration. There are two domains to the scale: one for consciousness and one for tolerance. There are two categories within the domain of consciousness (awakeness and comprehension) and three categories of tolerance (calmness, ventilator synchrony, and face relaxation). Behaviors are scored

Table 3
Motor Activity Assessment Scale

Score	Definition
0 Unresponsive	Does not move with noxious stimuli
1 Responsive only to noxious stimuli	Opens eyes or raises eyebrows or turns head toward stimulus or moves limbs with noxious stimuli
2 Responsive to touch or name	Opens eyes or raises eyebrows or turns head toward stimulus or moves limbs when touched or name is loudly spoken
3 Calm and cooperative	No external stimulus is required to elicit movement and patient adjusts sheets or clothes purposefully and follows commands
4 Restless and cooperative	No external stimulus is required to elicit movement and patient picks at sheets or tubes or uncovers self and follows commands
5 Agitated	No external stimulus is required to elicit movement and attempts to sit up or moves limbs out of bed and does not consistently follow commands (eg, lies down when asked but soon reverts back to attempts to sit up or move limbs out of bed)
6 Dangerously agitated, uncooperative	No external stimulus is required to elicit movement and patient pulls at tubes or catheters or thrashes side to side or strikes at staff or tries to climb out of bed and does not calm down when asked

From Devlin JW, Boleski G, Mlynarek M, et al. Motor Activity Assessment Scale: a valid and reliable sedation scale for use with mechanically ventilated patients in a adult surgical intensive care unit. Crit Care Med 1999;27:1271−5; with permission.

Table 4

The Vancouver Interaction and Calmness Scale

	Strongly agree	Agree	Mildly agree	Mildly disagree	Disagree	Strongly disagree
Interaction Score/30						
Patient interacts	6	5	4	3	2	1
Patient communicates	6	5	4	3	2	1
Information communicated by patient is reliable	6	5	4	3	2	1
Patient cooperates	6	5	4	3	2	1
Patient needs encouragement to respond to questions	1	2	3	4	5	6
Calmness score/30						
Patient appears calm	6	5	4	3	2	1
Patient appears restless	1	2	3	4	5	6
Patient appears distressed	1	2	3	4	5	6
Patient is moving around uneasily in bed	1	2	3	4	5	6
Patient is pulling at lines and tubes	1	2	3	4	5	6

Data from de Lemos J, Tweeddale M, Chittock D. Measuring quality of sedation in adult mechanically ventilated critically ill patients. J Clin Epidemiol 2000;53:908–19.

Table 5

The Richmond Agitation Scale

Score	Term	Description
+4	Combative	Overtly combative or violent, immediate danger to staff
+3	Very agitated	Pulls on or removes tubes or catheters or has aggressive behavior toward staff
+2	Agitated	Frequent nonpurposeful movement or patient-ventilator dyssynchrony
+1	Restless	Anxious or apprehensive but movements not aggressive or vigorous
0	Alert and calm	
−1	Drowsy	Not fully alert, but has sustained (more than 10 seconds) awakening, with eye contact, to voice
−2	Light sedation	Briefly (less than 10 seconds) awakens with eye to contact to voice
−3	Moderate sedation	Any movement (but no eye contact) to voice
−4	Deep sedation	No response to voice, but any movement to physical stimulation
−5	Unarousable	No response to voice or physical stimulation

From Sessler CN, Gosnell MS, Grap MJ, et al. The Richmond Agitation-Sedation Scale: validity and reliability in adult intensive care unit patients. Am J Respir Crit Care Med 2002;166:1338–44; with permission.

for each category (Table 6). The instrument has undergone interrater reliability and validity testing with several other scales, with favorable results [30]. The reader is referred to the citation for detailed information about testing of the scale.

Objective measures of sedation

Development of objective measures of sedation is needed to assist in achieving appropriate depth to avoid undersedation and oversedation. Bispectral index monitoring is a type of electroencephalogram, which is monitored with several electrodes attached to the forehead. The scale ranges from 0 (isoelectric electroencephalogram) to 100 (completely awake) and is derived from several electroencephalogram components including degree of suppression, relative power in several frequency ranges, and other bispectral elements [32]. A score of 60 corresponds to deep sedation and is commonly the range recommended in the ICU [33]. Bispectral index monitoring has demonstrated mixed results in studies reporting correlation with subjective scoring systems. The newer version bispectral index monitoring XP, however, has shown much stronger correlation with the RASS ($R^2 = .742$); Riker Sedation-Agitation-Scale ($R^2 = .742$); and Glasgow Coma Scale ($R^2 = .685$) [34].

Actigraphy may be useful in objectively evaluating sedation from the perspective of limb movement versus central nervous system level of wakefulness. The actigraph, which is placed on the wrist, senses and records movement detection and vigor over time. The device translates the movement detection to an electrical signal, which is continuously sampled by a

Table 6
The ATICE

Consciousness domain graded 0–5		Tolerance domain		
Awakeness	Comprehension, sum of 1 point responses	Calmness, graded 0–3	Ventilator synchrony, sum of 1 point elements	Face relaxation, graded 0–3
Eyes close, no mimic 0	Open/close eyes 1	Life-threatening agitation 0	No blockade of the inspiratory phase of ventilation 1	Permanent grimacing 0
Eyes closed, only face mimic after strong painful stimulation 1	Open your mouth 1	Agitation, does not respond to verbal order 1	No respiratory rate > 30 1	Severe provoked grimacing 1
Eyes open after strong painful stimulation 2	Look at me 1	Agitation, responds to verbal order 2	No cough 1	Moderate provoked grimacing 2
Eyes open after light painful stimulation 3	Nod yes with head 1	Calm 3	No use of accessory muscles 1	Relaxed face 3
Eyes open after verbal order 4	Close eyes and open mouth 1			
Eyes open spontaneously 5				

Data from De Jonghe BD, Cook D, Griffith L, et al. Adaptation to the intensive care environment (ATICE): development and validation of a new sedation assessment instrument. Crit Care Med 2003;31:2344–54.

microprocessor and stored in memory [35]. Validity, reliability, and sensitivity have been well established in the laboratory and in clinical research to discriminate between sedentary and nonsedentary activities [35,36]. It has been used to detect initial limb movement and vigor in an evaluation of recovery after termination of neuromuscular blockade in critically ill adults, showing strong correlation with a five-point muscle scoring system [37]. Actigraphy has also been used for detection of excessive limb movement as a measure of agitation caused by inadequate sedation. Validation was achieved through Spearman rho correlation coefficients of wrist and ankle actigraphy counts with the RASS and COMFORT scales, researcher observation of stimulation, and blood pressure and heart rate. Wrist actigraphy counts correlated with the RASS ($r = 0.58$) and COMFORT ($r = 0.62$) scales. Likewise, ankle actigraphy data correlated with RASS ($r = 0.52$) and COMFORT ($r = 0.48$) scales. Correlation with observed stimulation and blood pressure measures was modest; there was no correlation between actigraphy data and heart rate [38].

Refinement of methods to accurately evaluate patient level of sedation and achievement of sedation goals is needed. A comprehensive approach to include the reasons patients require sedation is needed to determine the effectiveness. Measures of oxygenation, heart rate, intracranial pressure in conjunction with anxiety measures, and reduction in agitation and physical activity provide necessary information to clinicians in determining whether or not the patient is at the right level of sedation. Recognizing and main-

taining the appropriate level without overshooting reduces complications of oversedation and contributes to more clinically beneficial and cost-effective patient outcomes.

Selection of sedative and method of administration

There are no published reports describing an ideal sedative for use in critically ill patients. Midazolam, lorazepam, propofol, diazepam, and a newer agent, dexmedetomidine, are described in the literature. In a double-blind, randomized, controlled study of 64 mechanically ventilated patients requiring support for more than 3 days, Swart and colleagues [39] compared lorazepam with midazolam for sedation effectiveness, dosing, and plasma levels. They found that sedation level was easier to reach with lorazepam and there was a significant cost savings. There were no differences in recovery, however, 24 hours after termination of either drug.

In contrast, other researchers demonstrated that a continuous infusion of midazolam was superior to lorazepam in achieving effective sedation and reducing costs. In a study of 58 patients, 27 received midazolam and 31 received lorazepam. Effective sedation was defined by Ramsay score 2 to 4 60% of the time; costs included the ICU and hospital stays, duration of mechanical ventilation, tracheostomy placement, and charges for opiates and benzodiazepines. They found that more patients achieved effective sedation in the midazolam group (77%) compared with the lorazepam group (45%, $P = .016$). Although not statistically significant, they found costs for the midazolam group were less ($19,895 ± 18,177 versus $22,081 ± 15,630 [$P = .624$] for the lorazepam group). Of greatest interest, the amount of time patients were oversedated (Ramsay score 5–6) was less in the midazolam group than the lorazepam group (18% versus 36%, $P = .009$) [21].

These findings are consistent with those from another study. Continuous infusions of lorazepam, midazolam, and propofol were compared in a prospective, randomized, nonblinded study of 30 mechanically ventilated patients. Sedation was initiated and maintained to achieve a Ramsay score between 2 and 5. Investigators determined that maintenance doses of lorazepam, midazolam, and propofol were achieved 68%, 79%, and 62% of the time during assessment, respectively. Oversedation was most often associated with lorazepam use compared with the other two drugs (15% versus 6% for midazolam and 7% for propofol). Mean sedation costs per patient day were $48 ± $76 for lorazepam, $182 ± $98 for midazolam, and $273 ± $200 for propofol ($P = .005$) [40]. This is an example of lower shelf costs for the medication that may be off-set by the costs of oversedation. In an earlier randomized, prospective study of mechanically ventilated patients, recovery of mental status was longer with midazolam (76 hours) than lorazepam (11 hours). Although the differences were not statistically significant, return to baseline mental status was much longer than anticipated [41].

Sedation administration by intravenous bolus injection versus continuous infusion may reduce the risk of oversedation and prolonged sedation. Kollef and coworkers [42] reported in a prospective observational study of 246 ICU patients who required mechanical ventilation that there was a significantly longer duration of mechanical ventilation with continuous infusion of sedation versus bolus administration or no intravenous sedation ($P \leq .001$). Shaw and colleagues [43] evaluated a semiautomated sedation infusion system in a study of 37 critically ill patients. They found that bolus injections of sedatives were effective in reducing mean agitation by 68.4% and peak agitation by 52.9%. Medication consumption differed from the recorded drug dose by 72.6% to 101%. The investigators concluded that using a semiautomated system reduces the risk of oversedation because less drug amount may be used to control agitation compared with delivery by continuous infusion.

Daily interruption of sedation is proposed to guard against oversedation and prevent prolonged sedative effects. One hundred twenty-eight patients were randomized to daily interruption of sedation or to sedation directed by the medical ICU team. In a blinded, retrospective review of the database of 128 patients, seven complications associated with critical illness and mechanical ventilation were identified: ventilator-associated pneumonia, upper gastrointestinal hemorrhage, bacteremia, barotraumas, venous thromboembolic events, cholestasis, and sinusitis. The investigators reviewed the records for incidence of these complications and found 13 complications (2.8%) in patients who had daily sedation interruption and 26 complications (6.2%) in patients in the control group ($P = .04$) [44]. Daily interruption of sedation may be beneficial in reducing complications of critical illness and mechanical ventilation.

Many clinicians prefer continuous infusion of intravenous sedation because it provides a more steady blood level and reduces the risk of dangerous breakthrough agitation between bolus doses. Continuous infusion may also be more nurse-time efficient, without the need for frequent bolus administration and associated procedures necessary for administration of a controlled substance. Steady blood levels, however, may be altered by inefficient drug metabolism and elimination processes associated with hepatic or renal dysfunction common to critical illness and actually result in higher rather than steady levels of sedation. This could, in turn, contribute to prolonged sedation effects. Furthermore, when one considers the reasons for administering sedation (ie, agitation, anxiety, facilitation of medical therapeutic regimen, ventilator tolerance and oxygenation, control of intracranial pressure, hemodynamic stability, and overall patient safety), drug holiday may be contraindicated in many critically ill individuals. Cessation of sedation may foster dangerous agitation, create oxygen supply and demand mismatch, and numerous other responses that negate other clinical management efforts. Drug holiday must be carefully evaluated using a risk-benefit model.

Summary

Sedation is a necessary aspect of managing critical illness. Control of agitation and anxiety to maximize the therapeutic management plan and promote healing are the overriding goals of sedation in the ICU. Oversedation negates many of the restorative processes, however, and contributes to multiple complications, including prolonged immobility and related complications, such as severe weakness. Critically ill patients have multiple etiologies for the development of severe weakness, as illustrated by the case example described at the beginning of this article. Oversedation acts synergistically with other risk factors and perpetuates a cycle of inactivity, muscle wasting, and extreme weakness. Oversedation increases ventilator days and prolongs length of ICU and hospital stay, which translates into exponential cost increases. Improved methods of evaluating appropriate levels of sedation, techniques in medication delivery, appropriate medication selection, and nonburdensome ways to assess muscle strength and integrity contribute to improved functional outcomes for patients following critical illness.

References

[1] Shafer A. Complications of sedation with midazolam in the intensive care unit and a comparison with other sedative regimens. Crit Care Med 1998;26:947–56.

[2] Hogarth DK, Hall J. Management of sedation in mechanically ventilated patients. Curr Opin Crit Care 2004;10:40–6.

[3] Barrientos-Vega R, Sanchez-Soria MM, Morales-Garcia C, et al. Prolonged sedation of critically ill patients with midazolam or propofol: impact on weaning and costs. Crit Care Med 1997;25:33–40.

[4] Winkelman C. Inactivity and inflammation: selected cytokines as biologic mediators in muscle dysfunction during critical illness. AACN Clin Issues 2004; 15:74–82.

[5] Zochdne DW, Ramsay D, Shelley S. Acute necrotizing myopathy of intensive care: electrophysiological studies. Muscle Nerve 1994;17:285–92.

[6] Bolton CF. Neuromuscular complications of sepsis. Intensive Care Med 1993;19:S58–63.

[7] Murray M, Cowen J, DeBlock H, et al. Clinical guidelines for sustained neuromuscular blockade in the adult critically ill patient. Crit Care Med 2002;30: 142–56.

[8] Latronico N. Neuromuscular alterations in the critically ill patient: critical illness myopathy, critical illness neuropathy, or both? Intensive Care Med 2003;29: 1411–3.

[9] Bolton CF, Gilbert JJ, Hahn AF, et al. Polyneuropathy in critically ill patients. J Neurol Neurosurg Psychiatry 1984;47:1223–31.

[10] Fletcher SN, Kennedy DD, Ghosh IR, et al. Persistent neuromuscular and neurophysiologic abnormalities in ling-term survivors of prolonged critical illness. Crit Care Med 2003;31:1012–6.

[11] Griffin DO, Fairman N, Coursin D, et al. Acute myopathy during treatment of status asthmaticus with corticosteroids and steroid muscle relaxants. Chest 1992;102:510–4.

[12] Bednarik J, Lukas Z, Vondracek P. Critical illness polyneuromyopathy: the electrophysiological components of a complex entity. Intensive Care Med 2003; 29:1505–14.

[13] Latronico N, Peli E, Botteri M. Critical illness myopathy and neuropathy. Curr Opin Crit Care 2005;11: 126–32.

[14] Al-Jumah MA, Awada AA, Al-Ayafi HA, et al. Neuromuscular paralysis in the intensive care unit. Saudi Med J 2004;25:474–7.

[15] Kasper C. Antecedent condition: impaired physical mobility. In: Metzger BL, editor. Altered functioning: impairment and disability. Indianapolis (IN): Nursing Center Press of Sigma Theta Tau International; 1991. p. 20–30.

[16] Greenleaf JE, Kozlowski S. Physiological consequences of reduced physical activity during bed rest. Exerc Sport Sci Rev 1982;10:84–119.

[17] Booth FW, Seider MJ. Early change in skeletal muscle protein synthesis after limb immobilization of rats. J Appl Physiol 1979;47:974–7.

[18] Kasper CE, Talbot LA, Gaines JM. Skeletal muscle damage and recovery. AACN Clin Issues 2002;13: 237–47.

[19] Booth FW. Time course of muscle atrophy during immobilization of hindlimbs in rats. J Appl Physiol 1977;43:656–61.

[20] Cernaianu AC, DelRossi AJ, Flum DR, et al. Lorazepam and midazolam in the intensive care unit: a randomized, prospective, multicenter study of hemodynamics, oxygen transport, efficacy, and cost. Crit Care Med 1996;24:222–8.

[21] Micek S, Barnes BJ, Johnson DC. Long-term sedation with protocol-directed midazolam and lorazepam: a cost effectiveness analysis. Crit Care Med 2004; 32(Suppl):A174.

[22] Carrasco G. Instruments for monitoring intensive care unit sedation. Crit Care 2000;4:217–25.

[23] Ramsay M, Savege T, Simpson BRJ, et al. Controlled sedation with alphaxalone/alphadolone. BMJ 1974; 2:656–9.

[24] Harris E, O'Donnell C, Macmillan RR, et al. Use of propofol infusion for sedation of patients undergoing haemofiltration: assessment of the effect of haemofiltration on the level of sedation on blood propofol concentration. J Drug Dev 1991;4(Suppl 3):37–9.

[25] Fraser GL, Riker R. Monitoring sedation, agitation, analgesia, and delirium in critically ill adult patients. Crit Care Clin 2001;17:1–21.

[26] Devlin JW, Boleski G, Mlynarek M, et al. Motor Activity Assessment Scale: a valid and reliable sedation scale for use with mechanically ventilated patients in a adult surgical intensive care unit. Crit Care Med 1999;27:1271–5.

[27] de Lemos J, Tweeddale M, Chittock D. Measuring quality of sedation in adult mechanically ventilated critically ill patients. J Clin Epidemiol 2000; 53:908–19.

[28] Ambuel B, Hamlett KW, Marx CM, et al. Assessing distress in pediatric intensive care environments: the COMFORT scale. J Pediatr Psychol 1992;17:95–109.

[29] Sessler CN, Gosnell MS, Grap MJ, et al. The Richmond Agitation-Sedation Scale: validity and

reliability in adult intensive care unit patients. Am J Respir Crit Care Med 2002;166:1338–44.

[30] De Jonghe BD, Cook D, Griffith L, et al. Adaptation to the intensive care environment (ATICE): development and validation of a new sedation assessment instrument. Crit Care Med 2003;31:2344–54.

[31] Riker RR, Fraser G, Cox PM. Continuous infusion haloperidol controls agitation in critically ill patients. Crit Care Med 1994;22:433–40.

[32] Rampil IJ. A primer for EEG signal processing in anesthesia. Anesthesiology 1998;89:980–1002.

[33] McGaffigan P. Advancing sedation assessment to promote patient comfort. Crit Care Nurse 2002;(Suppl):29–36.

[34] Deogaonkar A, Gupta R, De Georgia M, et al. Bispectral index monitoring correlates with sedation scales in brain-injured patients. Crit Care Med 2004;32:2403–6.

[35] Tryon WW. Activity measurement in psychology and medicine. New York: Plenum Press; 1991.

[36] Patterson SM, Krantz DS, Montgomery LC, et al. Automated physical activity monitoring: validation and comparison with physiological and self-report measures. Psychopathology 1993;30:296–305.

[37] Foster J. Functional recovery following neuromuscular blockade in critically ill adults [doctoral dissertation]. Austin (TX): The University of Texas at Austin; 2001.

[38] Grap MJ, Borchers T, Munro C, et al. Actigraphy in the critically ill: correlation with activity, agitation, and sedation. Am J Crit Care 2005;14:52–60.

[39] Swart EL, van Schijndel RJ, Loenen AC, et al. Continuous infusion of lorazepam versus midazolam in patients in the intensive care unit: sedation with lorazepam is easier to manage and is more cost-effective. Crit Care Med 1999;27:1461–5.

[40] McCollam JS, O'Neil MG, Norcross ED, et al. Continuous infusions of lorazepam, midazolam, and propofol for sedation of the critically ill surgery trauma patient: a prospective randomized comparison. Crit Care Med 1999;27:2454–8.

[41] Pohlman AS, Simpson KP, Hall JP. Continuous intravenous infusion of lorazepam versus midazolam for sedation during mechanical ventilatory support: a prospective randomized study. Crit Care Med 1994;22:1241–7.

[42] Kollef MH, Levy NT, Ahrens TS, et al. The use of continuous IV sedation is associated with prolongation of mechanical ventilation. Chest 1998;114:360–1.

[43] Shaw G, Rudge A, Hooper E, et al. Emerging methods for sedation and agitation management in critical illness. Crit Care Med 2004;32(Suppl):A97.

[44] Schweickert WD, Gehlbach BK, Pohlman AS, et al. Daily interruption of sedative infusions and complications of critical illness in mechanically ventilated patients. Crit Care Med 2004;32:1272–6.

ELSEVIER
SAUNDERS

Crit Care Nurs Clin N Am 17 (2005) 297–304

CRITICAL CARE
NURSING CLINICS
OF NORTH AMERICA

Alcohol Withdrawal Syndrome: Assessment and Treatment with the Use of the Clinical Institute Withdrawal Assessment for Alcohol-Revised

Carol A. Puz, RN, MS, CCRN*, Sandra J. Stokes, RN, MSN

The Western Pennsylvania Hospital, 4800 Friendship Avenue, Pittsburgh, PA, 15224, USA

Alcohol consumption is part of American culture and is an acceptable part of social activities, an expected and anticipated part of college life, and an integral part of holiday preparations. Common psychosocial benefits of drinking alcohol include increased sociability, relaxation, stress reduction, and mood elevation [1–4]. In fact, 44% of adults in the United States ages 18 and over have consumed at least 12 drinks in the preceding year [5]. According to the United States Department of Agriculture and the United States Department of Health and Human Services, moderate drinking is no more than two standard drinks per day for men and no more than one drink per day for women. In the United States, a drink is considered to be 0.5 oz of alcohol, which is equivalent to 12 oz of beer, 5 oz of wine, or 1.5 oz of 80-proof distilled spirits [6].

When alcohol is abused, it can have an impact on human behavior, leading to property damage, legal problems, disruption in family relationships, interruption of academic achievements, and destruction of productive careers. Alcohol is the most widely available addictive drug in America, is a known toxin, and has negative effects on virtually every organ in the human body [7]. Approximately 77% of the annual $185 billion cost of alcohol misuse is health related, generated by medical consequences and lost productivity associated with illness or death

[8]. Alcohol-related illness and injury account for at least 8% of all emergency department visits [9].

Abuse and dependence

Alcohol abuse can be defined as when individuals drink despite alcohol-related physical, social, psychologic, or occupational consequences or when in dangerous situations, such as operating machinery or a motor vehicle. Alcohol dependence, also known as alcoholism, includes physiologic symptoms, such as tolerance (the need to drink greater amounts to elicit the same effect); behavioral symptoms, such as a strong urge to drink (craving) and not being able to stop drinking once drinking has started; and withdrawal symptoms, such as nausea, diaphoresis, tremors, and anxiety after the cessation of drinking [10].

Effects of alcohol on system function

Alcohol is soluble in water and fat, so it is distributed rapidly to all body tissues and crosses the blood-brain barrier easily, exerting its intoxicating effects on the brain [7]. When alcohol is consumed, approximately 20% of the alcohol is absorbed in the stomach and the remaining 80% is absorbed in the proximal small intestine. Beer and sparkling wines are carbonated, increasing the rate of absorption of

* Corresponding author.
E-mail address: cpuz@wpahs.org (C.A. Puz).

alcohol [7]. Food delays gastric emptying and consequently delays the rate of alcohol absorption in the body, because the alcohol takes longer to reach the small intestine.

Alcohol has many acute and chronic effects on multiple organ systems. The systems affected most commonly are the gastrointestinal (GI) system and the central nervous system (CNS). Damage from chronic alcohol use also can occur in the cardiovascular, genitourinary, and hematopoietic systems.

Repeated consumption of alcohol in large quantities can damage the GI system as alcohol breaks down the protective mucus barrier of the stomach, leading to gastritis and bleeding. Alcohol can cause esophagitis, Mallory-Weiss lesions, and esophageal varices. Alcohol use also can lead to malnutrition. The empty calories in alcohol suppress the appetite. Malnutrition leads to thiamine deficiency, which impairs cellular metabolism in all tissues [11]. Disruption in vitamin absorption and use occurs with chronic alcohol consumption. Deterioration of liver function is a GI consequence of excessive alcohol consumption. Alcoholic liver disease is the second leading diagnosis precipitating the need for liver transplantation [5]. In the liver, alcohol is converted to acetaldehyde. Acetaldehyde initiates hepatic changes, which include fat deposition, liver enlargement, and the destruction of hepatocytes, resulting in the development of cirrhosis [11]. Hepatitis and pancreatitis, associated with alcohol abuse and dependence, are consequences of acetaldehyde exposure.

Alcohol affects the CNS in a variety of ways. Alcohol's acute effect on the CNS includes impaired judgment, motor coordination, balance, and reaction time. Alcohol is a depressant. In low doses, it causes acute effects by depressing inhibitory synapses, resulting in giddiness, euphoria, and enhanced confidence [7]. Alcohol subsequently depresses excitatory synapses, however, which results in relaxation and drowsiness. It even may produce coma and death when blood alcohol levels reach levels of 400 mg/dL [7]. Chronic effects of repeated consumption of alcohol in large quantities can lead to brain disorders, such as Korsakoff's psychosis (a result of thiamine deficiency), dementia, loss of cognitive function, and brain atrophy [12].

The cardiovascular system is affected when liver function is impaired. The liver cannot synthesize clotting factors and blood clotting is impaired. Edema results from inadequate synthesis of blood albumin. Portal hypertension results when the cirrhotic liver obstructs the hepatic portal blood circulation. The combination of portal hypertension and decreased albumin levels causes the liver and other organs to leak serous fluid into the peritoneal cavity. The abdomen then can become edematous and ascites develops. Impaired clotting mechanisms, in conjunction with portal hypertension and esophageal varices, increase the risk of hemorrhage. Alcohol abuse and the consequent thiamine deficiency impair myocardial cell metabolism, which reduces contractile strength of the heart and leads to the development of heart failure [11].

Alcohol affects the genitourinary system in multiple ways. In men, excess alcohol consumption can lead to erectile dysfunction and testicular atrophy. In women, amenorrhea, spontaneous abortion, and fetal abnormalities can occur [10].

Chronic alcohol abuse and dependence can lead to bone disorders, alcoholic myopathy, and immune suppression, leading to recurrent infection. They are also implicated as risk factors in the development of breast cancer [10].

Alcohol withdrawal syndrome

Approximately 8.2 million people, including an estimated 15% to 20% of all primary care and hospitalized patients, are dependent on alcohol [13,14]. Alcohol withdrawal syndrome (AWS) can occur when alcohol consumption is reduced or stopped. Alcohol depresses neuronal excitability and impulse conduction. When the brain no longer is exposed to alcohol, brain hyperexcitability results, which leads to the development of the symptoms of AWS [15]. Symptoms of AWS are affected by the amount of alcohol consumed and the duration of the drinking habit [15]. Symptoms of AWS can begin several hours after the blood alcohol levels decline and symptoms peak during the second day of abstinence [16,17].

Minor withdrawal symptoms can appear 6 to 12 hours after abstinence from alcohol. These symptoms include insomnia, tremors, mild anxiety, GI upset, headache, diaphoresis, palpitations, and anorexia. Approximately 7% of patients who have AWS develop alcoholic hallucinosis [10]. These symptoms occur 12 to 24 hours after the cessation of alcohol consumption. The symptoms include visual, auditory, or tactile hallucinations. Between 5% and 10% of patients develop tonic-clonic withdrawal seizures approximately 24 to 48 hours after alcohol is stopped [10]. The development of seizures increases as the number of withdrawal episodes patients have experienced in the past increases, even if the episodes were managed medically [10].

Delirium tremens

Approximately 5% of patients who have AWS progress to a more severe form of AWS known as delirium tremens (DT). This syndrome develops most frequently within 2 to 4 days of withdrawal from alcohol. Symptoms during this time include hallucinations, disorientation, hypertension, tachycardia, low-grade fever, diaphoresis, increased respiratory rate, and agitation. The development of DT is viewed as a medical emergency leading to respiratory and cardiovascular collapse and death. This condition has a mortality rate of 1% to 5% [16]. Factors that increase the likelihood of developing DT include pre-existing medical illness, abnormal liver function, daily heavy alcohol use, older age, and previous history of DT or withdrawal seizures [15].

Patient assessment

Critical to the timely initiation of treatment of alcohol withdrawal is an accurate history of alcohol intake. Wherever the admission—emergency department, general medical or surgical unit, intensive care unit, telemetry or step-down unit, or outpatient setting—the assessment for withdrawal from alcohol must be initiated. Before using an assessment tool, interviewers must assess the quantity, frequency, and pattern of alcohol intake. Patients and families often are reluctant to discuss the use of alcohol. Because the description of alcohol quantity consumed can be subjective [18], accurate assessments can be a challenge. People do not come forth and announce the need for treatment of alcoholism; rather, the signs must be recognized. Questions such as "How many drinks do you consume per week?" or "What is the maximum number of drinks per occasion?" may give needed clues to detecting alcoholism. Generally, for men, more than 14 drinks per week or more than 4 per occasion, and for women, more than 7 drinks per week or more than 3 per occasion are signs of possible abuse or dependence [19].

A widely used assessment tool is the CAGE questionnaire [20]. It consists of four questions useful in the diagnosing of alcoholism. CAGE is easy for interviewers to recall: cutting down, annoyance by criticism, guilty feelings, and eye-opener [21]. The questions are

1. Have you ever felt you should cut down on your drinking?
2. Have people annoyed you by criticizing your drinking?

3. Have you ever felt bad or guilty about your drinking?
4. Have you ever had an eye-opener drink first thing in the morning to steady your nerves or to get rid of a hangover?

Answers are scored as 0 for no and 1 for yes. Patients who have a score of 2 or higher require a more detailed assessment for alcohol withdrawal [20].

Assessment of the signs and symptoms of alcohol withdrawal that indicate autonomic hyperactivity is performed best with a standardized assessment tool for scoring symptoms [18]. The revised Clinical Institute Withdrawal Assessment for Alcohol scale (CIWA-Ar) is the tool used most widely for assessing alcohol withdrawal. It measures nine categories of symptoms on a scale of 0 to 7 and one symptom (clouding sensorium) on a scale of 0 to 4. Mild symptoms translate into a total score of less than 8, moderate symptoms 8 to15, and severe symptoms greater than 15. Patients who have a score of greater than or equal to 8 should receive drug therapy to treat their symptoms and reduce the risk of seizures and DT.

The tool is not copyrighted and can be reproduced freely. It is a way of quantifying alcohol withdrawal syndrome. Quantification is key to preventing excess morbidity and mortality in a group of patients who are at risk for alcohol withdrawal [23]. The tool allows for appropriate pharmacotherapy intervention. By quantifying and monitoring the withdrawal process, treatment regimens can be adjusted to meet the needs of individual patients (Fig. 1). Protocols then can be established to guide nurses and physicians regarding the administration of medications. Scores of less than 8 to 10 may indicate minimal to mild withdrawal, scores of 8 to 15 may indicate moderate withdrawal (marked autonomic arousal), and scores of 15 or more may indicate severe withdrawal (impending DT) [22]. The higher the score, the greater the risk for severe alcohol withdrawal. Despite low scores, if left untreated, complications can occur. An example of an alcohol detoxification protocol can be found in Box 1.

Clinical management

Psychologic and medication treatments are two approaches that complement each other in attaining successful and effective treatment outcomes [24]. A consultation with a psychiatric/addiction specialist is necessary to determine the presence of any coexisting psychiatric illness. Recovery-focused treatment

Patient:	Date:	Time:

Heart Rate (taken for one minute):	Blood Pressure:

CATEGORY	RANGE OF SCORES	SCORING EXAMPLES
Agitation Observation	0 - 7	0 = normal activity 4 = moderately fidgety and restless 7 = constantly trashes about
Anxiety Ask, "Do you feel nervous?"	0 - 7	0 = no anxiety, at ease 4 = moderately anxious or guarded 7 = acute panic state
Auditory disturbances Ask, "Are you more aware of sounds around you? Are they harsh? Do they frighten you? Are you hearing anything that is disturbing to you? Are you hearing things you know are not there?"	0 - 7	0 = not present 4 = moderately severe hallucinations 7 = continuous hallucinations
Clouding of sensorium Ask, "What day is it? Where are you? Who am I?"	0 - 4	0 = oriented and can do serial additions 2 = disoriented for date by no more than two calendar days 4 = disoriented for place and/or person
Headache Ask, "Does your head feel different? Does it feel like there is a band around your head?" Do not rate for dizziness or lightheadedness. Otherwise, rate severity.	0 - 7	0 = not present 4 = moderately severe 7 = extremely severe
Nausea or vomiting Ask, "Do you feel sick to your stomach? Have you vomited"?	0 - 7	0 = no nausea and no vomiting 4 = intermittent nausea and dry heaves 7 = constant nausea, frequent dry heaves and vomiting
Paroxysmal sweats	0 - 7	0 = no sweat visible 4 = beads of sweat obvious on forehead 7 = drenching sweats
Tactile disturbances Ask, "Have you any itching, pins and needles sensations, any burning, any numbness, or do you feel bugs crawling on or under your skin?"	0 - 7	0 = none 4 = moderately severe hallucinations 7 = continuous hallucinations
Tremor Arms extended and fingers spread apart.	0 - 7	0 = no tremor 4 = moderate with patient's arm extended 7 = severe even without extended arms
Visual disturbances Ask, "Does the light appear to be too bright? Is its color different? Does it hurt your eye? Are you seeing anything that is disturbing to you? Are you seeing things you know are not there?"	0 - 7	0 = none 4 = moderately severe hallucinations 7 = continuous hallucinations

TOTAL SCORE: _____   RATER'S INITIALS: _____

Fig. 1. Revised Clinical Institute Withdrawal Assesment of Alcohol.

Box 1. Using the revised Clinical Institute Withdrawal Assessment of Alcohol Scale in a protocol

1. Physician orders CIWA-Ar protocol.
2. CIWA-Ar completed on admission and every 8 hours for 24 hours. Vital signs every shift. Document CIWA-Ar and vital signs on nursing flow sheet located in the chart. If CIWA-Ar is ≤8 times 3, discontinue CIWA-Ar protocol.
3. If CIWA-Ar is >0 but <8 and vital signs are stable, no medication is required. Repeat vital signs every 4 hours and CIWA-Ar every 8 hours.
4. If CIWA-Ar is >8 but <15, or diastolic blood pressure is >110, give lorazepam 2 mg by mouth or intramuscularly and repeat CIWA-Ar in 8 hours. Vital signs every 4 hours.
5. If CIWA-Ar is >15 or diastolic blood pressure is >110, give lorazepam 2 mg by mouth or intramuscularly every 1 hour until patient has CIWA-Ar <15. CIWA and blood pressure checked every 1hour. If CIWA-Ar is between 8 and 15, give lorazepam 2 mg by mouth or intramuscularly and resume CIWA-Ar every 8 hours and vital signs every 4 hours.
6. Call physician if patient requires >6 mg of lorazepam in 3 hours.

From CBHA clinical practice guidelines: alcohol detoxification. Available at: http://www.cbhallc.com/exhibitf.html. Accessed December 1, 2004.

---

includes community-based mutual help groups, low-intensity outpatient treatment programs, high-intensity outpatient treatment programs, family or relationship therapy, individual therapy with a cognitive or behavioral focus, or residential treatment. A 12-step group program, such as Alcoholics Anonymous, with as individualized and comprehensive treatment program as patients can tolerate and afford, is optimal [15].

Medications for alcohol dependence can be used to accomplish specific goals, such as promoting abstinence or reducing heavy drinking, and medi-

cations can help patients achieve these goals by reducing the craving or the desire for alcohol, reducing the rewarding effects of alcohol, or reducing prolonged withdrawal symptoms [25]. Patients can benefit from supportive measures, such as quiet environments, reduced lighting, limited interactions with others, nutrition and fluids, and reassurance and encouragement [26].

The most commonly used medications include the benzodiazepines, such as chlordiazepoxide, diazepam, and lorazepam. These medications are recommended over others because they have better documented efficacy, are safer, and are less likely to lead to abuse [14]. Diazepam and chlordiazepoxide are long-acting agents that make withdrawal smoother and rebound withdrawal symptoms less likely to occur [15]. Lorazepam and oxazepam are intermediate-acting medications and may be the preferred agents in patients who metabolize medications less effectively, particularly the those who are elderly or who have liver failure [15]. One common mistake among clinicians is the undertreatment of alcohol withdrawal because of the reluctance to administer high doses of medications that may be necessary for symptom management.

The benzodiazepine medications are used to replace the alcohol depressant effects on the CNS [20]. This replacement counteracts the autonomic hyperactivity displayed with alcohol withdrawal. In addition, benzodiazepines and alcohol have similar effects on the brain and are described as cross tolerant; meaning that one agent can serve as a substitute for the other [17]. Because untreated or undertreated alcohol withdrawal can be fatal, prompt treatment and intervention are crucial [27,28]. By using the CIWA-Ar tool, consistency in patient management can be accomplished through a symptom-triggered approach. By using a protocol that regulates medication dosing, the risks of overmedicating or undermedicating for symptoms of withdrawal are decreased.

Symptom-triggered therapy can be initiated in any patient who has a history of consistent alcohol intake or a positive response to the CAGE questions. By implementing protocols based on the CIWA-Ar, nurses are directed to administer the prescribed medications. As the severity of the symptoms progresses, the medication dose increases. Nurses play a pivotal role in monitoring and scoring patients according to the protocol and administering medications as determined by the CIWA-Ar score. A consistent approach is necessary to successful patient outcomes. Lack of understanding about patients who have an addictive disorder can lead to a lack of objective judgment toward patients and their symptoms.

The goal in managing alcohol withdrawal is to minimize adverse outcomes (patient discomfort, seizures, delirium, and mortality) and to avoid the adverse effects of withdrawal medications, such as excess sedation. Two approaches that are identified are fixed dosing versus symptom management by using the CIWA-Ar tool. Use of individualized regimens with the tool is shown to reduce the amount of medication needed and the duration of treatment without differences in other outcomes, such as incidence of seizures or delirium [14,17]. Critical care monitoring may be indicated to manage alcohol withdrawal delirium, especially with high doses of benzodiazepines.

One study [22] suggests that for patients admitted to general medical services who experience alcohol withdrawal, symptom-triggered treatment is associated with a reduced risk of DT. This reduction in risk is observed as a significantly lower rate of DT, particularly in patients who had no prior documented episode of DT. Another study [22] reports less benzodiazepine use in a general hospital setting for patients admitted with alcohol dependency and managed with symptom-triggered therapy compared with usual care, but there was no reported difference in withdrawal complications. Other investigators [17] demonstrate that a symptom-triggered approach results in decreased duration of benzodiazepine use and increased rates of observation without pharmacologic therapy compared with a fixed-schedule strategy.

Adjunctive agents

There are several medications that can be helpful in the treatment of AWS. These medications should be used in conjunction with the benzodiazepines.

Haloperidol can be used to treat agitation and hallucinations, but it can lower the seizure threshold [15]. The use of atenolol, a β-blocker that blunts the sympathetic response, resulting in a slower heart rate and reduced oxygen consumption, in combination with oxazepam is shown to stabilize neuroexcitation and restore hemodynamic stability more quickly and to reduce alcohol craving more effectively than the use of oxazepam alone [15]. Adjunctive treatment with a β-blocker should be considered in patients who have coronary artery disease, who may not be able to tolerate the effects that alcohol withdrawal place on the cardiovascular system [26]. Clonidine also is shown to improve the autonomic symptoms of withdrawal [14]. Although phenytoin does not treat withdrawal seizures, it is an appropriate adjunct in patients who have an underlying seizure disorder [15].

On the horizon

Two drugs recently approved by the Food and Drug Administration for use in persons who are alcohol dependent are disulfiram and naltrexone [25]. Disulfiram was introduced as an aversive therapy for alcohol dependence; however, clinical trails find that it has inconsistent therapeutic value [25]. Patients who take disulfiram and drink alcohol experience an increased dilation of the arterial and capillary tone, which causes hypotension, nausea, vomiting, flushing, headache, and possibly palpitations, convulsions, and even death [25]. Patients must champion its use. Disulfiram may reduce drinking days in alcohol-dependent patients, but there is only minimal evidence that it facilitates abstinence [29]. Successful treatment with disulfiram is associated with clients reporting a stable home life, being married, taking the medication under direct supervision, and having contingencies requiring use (eg, loss of driver's license) [25].

Naltrexone has been studied extensively for alcohol dependence since the early 1990s. It reduces the desire for alcohol after drinking has been stopped. It acts by interfering with the actions of key brain chemicals called endogenous opioids [30]. By blocking the actions of endogenous opioids, naltrexone prevents alcohol from exerting its pleasant effects and may reduce patients' desire to drink [30].

Clinical trials are ongoing to evaluate additional medication approaches to alcoholism treatment. Medications that target brain chemicals, such as serotonin, are being tested [30]. The use of antidepressants is under investigation to determine if their use could induce changes in drinking behaviors [30]. The goal of pharmacotherapy is to achieve long-term abstinence from alcohol consumption.

Summary

Early identification of potential withdrawal from alcohol is key to successful patient outcomes. Screening through a careful history and use of standardized questionnaires, such as the CAGE and the CIWA-Ar, allows for prevention and early treatment of complications. Researchers continue to explore medication therapy that could redirect the course of treatment of alcoholism, including the psychosocial treatments that could best be used with specific drug therapies. In addition, subtypes of alcoholics and appropriate treatment are under investigation. Subtypes are identified as youth (ages 18 to 25) and genetic predisposition

[31]. Youth and adolescence provide a critical window of opportunity. The earlier alcohol use begins, the greater the likelihood of alcoholism [31]. Genes are responsible for approximately half of the risk for alcoholism, making it one of the most inheritable complex disorders [31]. Preventing early onset alcoholism has potential for far-reaching, long-term effects.

The National Institute on Alcohol Abuse and Alcoholism (NIAAA) has set forth a 5-year strategic plan to guide them in research. Because alcoholism now is accepted as a medical disorder, the focus on alcohol research has sharpened [31]. NIAAA's strategic plan identifies seven goals:

1. Identify genes that are involved in alcohol-associated disorders.
2. Identify mechanisms associated with neuro-adaptation at multiple levels of analysis (molecular, cellular, neural circuits, and behavior).
3. Identify additional science-based preventive interventions for use in specific circumstances, such as pregnancy and college-age drinking.
4. Further delineate biologic mechanisms involved in biomedical consequences associated with excessive alcohol consumption.
5. Develop medications that diminish craving for alcohol, reduce the likelihood of post-treatment relapse, and accelerate recovery of alcohol-damaged organs.
6. Advance knowledge of the influence of environment on expression of genes involved in alcohol-associated behavior, including the vulnerable adolescent years and special populations.
7. Further elucidate the relationship between alcohol and violence [31].

Each goal has key objectives identified and is supported by core strategies that will lead to development of programs, strategic initiatives, and specific actions that the NIAAA will pursue to achieve its mission.

References

[1] Baum-Baicker C. The psychological benefits of moderate alcohol consumption: a review of the literature. Drug Alcohol Depend 1985;15:305–22.
[2] Hauge R, Irgens-Jensen O. The experiencing of positive consequences of drinking in four Scandinavian countries. Br J Addict 1990;85:645–53.
[3] Leigh BC, Stacy AW. On the scope of alcohol expectancy research: remaining issues of measurement and meaning. Psychol Bull 1991;110:147–54.
[4] Makela K, Mustonen H. Positive and negative experiences related to drinking as a function of annual alcohol intake. Br J Addict 1988;83:403–8.
[5] Health risks and benefits of alcohol consumption. Alcohol Res Health 2000;24:3–4.
[6] US Department of Agriculture and US Department of Health and Human Services. Home and garden bulletin no. 232. 4th edition. Washington, DC: US Department of Agriculture; 1995.
[7] Saladin K. Alcohol and alcoholism. In: Kane KT, editor. Anatomy and physiology: the unity of form and function. Boston: McGraw-Hill; 1998. p. 957–8.
[8] Department of Health and Human Services statement by Ting-Kai Li, M.D., Director, National Institute on Alcohol Abuse and Alcoholism on fiscal year 2005. President's Budget Request for the National Institute on Alcohol Abuse and Alcoholism. Available at: http://www.niaaa.nih.gov/about/statement04.htm. Accessed November 29, 2004.
[9] McDonald III AJ, Wang N, Camargo Jr CA. US emergency department visits for alcohol-related diseases and injuries between 1992 and 2000. Arch Intern Med 2004;164:531–7.
[10] Compton P. Caring for the alcohol dependent patient. Nursing 2002;32:58–63.
[11] McCance K, Huether S. Alteration of cardiovascular function. In: Schrefer S, editor. Pathophysiology: the biologic basis for disease in adults and children. 2nd edition. St. Louis: Mosby; 1994. p. 1000–84.
[12] Longnecker G. How alcohol works. In: Perry VH, editor. How drugs work: drug abuse and the human body. Emeryville (CA): Ziff-Davis; 1994. p. 39–43.
[13] Substance Abuse and Mental Health Services Administration. Table 5.1A—substance dependence for specific substances in the past year, by age group: numbers in thousands, 2002. National survey on drug use and health. Available at: www.samhsa.gov/oasnhsda/2k2nsduh/2k2TabsCover.pdf. Accessed Nov. 18, 2003.
[14] Mayo-Smith MF, Cushman P, Hill A, et al. Pharmacological management of alcohol withdrawal: a meta-analysis and evidence-based practice guideline. JAMA 1997;278:144–51.
[15] Bayard M, McIntyre J, Hill K, et al. Alcohol withdrawal syndrome. Am Fam Physician 2004;69:1443–50.
[16] Kasser C, Geller A, Howell E, et al. Detoxification: principles and protocols. American Society of Addiction and Medicine. http://www.asam.org/pub1/detoxification.htm.
[17] Saitz R. Introduction to alcohol withdrawal. Alcohol Health Res World 1998;22:5–12.
[18] Mckay A, Koranda A, Axen D. Using a symptom-triggered approach to manage patients in acute alcohol withdrawal. Medsurg Nurs 2004;13:15–21.
[19] Tomaselli K. Asking about alcohol: what doctors need to find out. AMNEWS: March 15, 2004. Available at: http://www.ama-assn.org/amednews/2004/03/15/hlsa0315.htm. Accessed November 4, 2004.

[20] Ewing JA. Detecting alcoholism: the CAGE question-
     naire. JAMA 1984;252:1905–7.
[21] Mayfield D, McLeod G, Hall P. The CAGE question-
     naire: validation of a new alcoholism treatment. Am J
     Psychiatry 1974;131:1121–3.
[22] Sullivan J, Sykora K, Schneiderman J, et al. Assess-
     ment of alcohol withdrawal: the revised clinical
     institute withdrawal assessment for alcohol scale
     (CIWA-Ar). BrJ Addictions 1989;84:1353–7.
[23] American Society of Addiction and Medicine News,
     supplement (January–February), 2001.
[24] O'Malley S, Jaffe A, et al. Naltrexone and coping skills
     for alcohol dependence. Arch Gen Psychiatry 1992;49:
     881–7.
[25] Kenna G, Swift R. Pharmacotherapies for alcohol
     dependence. US Pharmacist 2004:93–101.
[26] Myrick H, Anton R. Treatment of alcohol withdrawal.
     Alcohol Health Res World 1998;22:38–43.

[27] Jarque-Lopez A, Gonzales-Reimers E, Rodriguez-
     Moreno F, et al. Prevalence and mortality of heavy
     drinkers in a general medical hospital unit. Alcohol
     Alcohol 2001;36:335–8.
[28] Jaeger T, Lohr R, Pankratz VS. Symptom-triggered
     therapy for alcohol withdrawal syndrome in medical
     inpatients. Mayo Clinic Procedure 2001;77:695–701.
[29] Garbutt JC, West SL. Pharmacological treatment of
     alcohol dependence: a review of the evidence. JAMA
     1999;281:1318–25.
[30] Fuller R, Hiller-Sturmhofel S. Alcoholism treatment in
     the United States: an overview. Alcohol Res Health
     1999;23:69–77.
[31] The National Institute on Alcohol Abuse and Al-
     coholism Strategic Plan. Available at: http://www.
     niaaa.nih.gov/about/stratext.htm. Accessed Novem-
     ber 29, 2004.

ELSEVIER
SAUNDERS

Crit Care Nurs Clin N Am 17 (2005) 305–309

CRITICAL CARE
NURSING CLINICS
OF NORTH AMERICA

Index

Note: Page numbers of article titles are in **boldface** type.

0899-5885/05/$ – see front matter © 2005 Elsevier Inc. All rights reserved.
doi:10.1016/S0899-5885(05)00066-3

ccnursing.theclinics.com

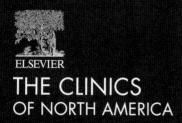